# Comments on Asthma – the 'at your fingertips' guide
## *from readers*

'Having asthma should not stop you leading a full and active life. With knowledge of my condition, the correct treatment and a desire to succeed, I became the Olympic champion.

This book gives you the knowledge. Don't limit yourself.'

*Adrian Moorhouse, MBE, Olympic Gold Medallist*

'This book provides the information necessary for those with asthma (and for those who live with those with asthma) to take control of their condition.'

*Dr Martyn Partridge, Chief Medical Adviser,*
*Asthma UK*

'This book is essential reading for both people with asthma and their doctors. It is easy to understand, and clearly and simply explains the different treatments now available for asthma.

Asthma sufferers and anyone involved in their care will find it of great benefit.'

*Dr Caroline Sykes, General Practitioner, London*

'I had the book bought as a Christmas present and I could not put it down. If I was not reading it my Dad was. Along with good pictures and clear information I really felt that somebody out there was listening to what asthmatics go through.

The book has given me great confidence and I feel that I am able to do more things than before.'

*Mrs Debbie Clarke, Birmingham*

'Your book was a pleasure to read: a clear, concise, informative account of the causes, symptoms, treatment and partial prevention of asthmatic conditions. I am glad I chose it amongst all the others available.'

*A. Roberts, Surrey*

'It is the best book I have read on asthma and the medication required to control it. Certainly a lot of research had gone into writing the book and I would like you to pass on our best wishes to the authors involved.'

*Ja*

D0676022

## Comments from readers (continued)

'I am pleased to be able to recommend it highly for patients with asthma and all who are involved in their care.'

*Professor E.D. Bateman, Respiratory Clinic,*
*Groote Schuur Hospital, South Africa*

'. . . I devoured your book.' – *C. Thornberry, South Africa*

'I have learnt so much more from your book than I have from the medical profession. You have changed my attitude towards my asthma, to look at it as taking control over it and not letting it dominate my life.'

*Mrs Penny Alderwick, Bristol*

'It certainly contains a lot of information which will undoubtedly help patients understand and cope with their disease. I shall be more than happy to recommend this book.'

*Dr Michael Rudolf, Consultant Physician,*
*Ealing Hospital NHS Trust*

'The authors are to be congratulated for making a very complex situation very understandable.'

*Professor Clive Page, Biomedical Sciences Division,*
*King's College London*

'I think it is an excellent book and one that will be very helpful.'

*Professor Richard Beasley, Professor of Medicine,*
*Wellington School of Medicine, New Zealand*

'Answers in a clear and readily understood fashion the questions that my patients ask and need information on. The format is simple and accessible.'

*Dr David Bellamy, General Practitioner, Bournemouth*

'An important contribution for asthma sufferers. It also provides support for health professionals.'

*Dr M.D.L. Morgan, Glenfield Hospital NHS Trust, Leicester*

'Extremely helpful, simply and well written.'

*Dr G. Skadding, Consultant Physician,*
*Royal National Throat Nose and Ear Hospital*

# Reviews of previous editions

'*Asthma at your fingertips* explains what causes asthma and gives a detailed explanation of the treatments available, guiding the reader through the complex world of inhalers, steroids and asthma clinics. The book devotes a whole chapter to children – from giving inhalers to babies to how best a child can cope at school – as well as looking at the way asthma can affect different areas of life, from pregnancy to work and even sex.'

*Essentials*

'. . . The book is written as a self-care manual, divided into sections such as what is asthma, issues to do with treatment, monitoring, coping in everyday life, and in emergencies, the needs of children, self help and complementary therapies. The book is organised around questions and answers. The success of this technique is in its clarity. The authors have provided enough information at a level that avoids being patronising. Surprisingly enough it is also very readable and avoids jargon and dense or medical writing. There is a sensitivity, but also an honesty about the limits of professional knowledge. There is a very useful glossary and index and list of addresses.'

*District Nursing Association Newsletter*

'This book will be welcomed by asthmatics, their relatives, and the many health professionals who are often asked to recommend a book. The authors are to be congratulated on the comprehensive contents, clear layout and the ease with which the book can be used . . . This book is well thought out and has been put together with the utmost care. It is a very useful addition to any asthmatic's and health professional's bookshelf.'

*Practice Nursing*

'Although most general practitioners will only learn a little from this book, I doubt there will be any general practitioner who will learn nothing. It is of special interest to those running asthma clinics, their nurses and patients.'

*Therapeutics Update*

# Reviews (continued)

'This new publication on asthma is undoubtedly excellent value for money, particularly for those who suffer from asthma or for parents of children who are affected.

Despite the book being aimed at this audience, it certainly has a place in the nursing and medical libraries, to complement the wealth of literature on the subject.

The book is logically presented and amusingly illustrated with cartoons. Clear diagrams are incorporated into the text and . . . information has been provided largely on a 'question and answer' basis, applying technical terminology which has been consistently and coherently explained. Chapters are also included on non-medical treatments and self help groups for people with asthma. Essentially, this is a comprehensive and practical guide to prevention, control and treatment of asthma which would be beneficial to sufferers, families, nurses and doctors.'

*Nursing Standard*

'I feel that this book is a great step forward in giving information to clients and is an essential reference for all health centres and public libraries. Even I, as someone who knows about and lives with the disease, picked up a few helpful ideas from this book and can highly recommend it to anyone involved in patient education about asthma and for those who suffer with asthma.'

*Nursing Times*

'This book may be considered one of the most valuable, comprehensive and readable of its kind. It is highly recommended for all patients who can be persuaded to learn more about their illness and embark on a programme of self management. All who care for patients with asthma are also advised to have one on their shelves.'

*South African Medical Journal*

'This [book] benefits from being presented in a question-and-answer format and offers an excellent judgement on all the things you had meant to ask your GP but never got round to.'

*Asthma News*

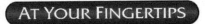

# ASTHMA

**Mark L Levy** MBChB, FRCGP
*General Practitioner, Harrow; Editor, GPIAG and Primary Care
Respiratory Journal; Clinical Research Fellow, Division of
Community Health Sciences: GP Section, University of Edinburgh;
and Medical Adviser, Education for Health, Warwick*

**Trisha Weller** MHS, RN
*Senior Module Leader and Programme Leader
BSc & Dip HE Respiratory Care, Education for Health, Warwick;
Asthma Nurse Specialist (Honorary Appt), Respiratory Department,
Birmingham Children's Hospital*

**Professor Sean Hilton** MD, FRCGP
*Professor of Primary Care and Head of Community
Health Sciences, Vice-Principal (Teaching and Learning)
St George's, University of London*

CLASS PUBLISHING • LONDON

Typography © Class Publishing
Fourth edition text © Mark Levy, Trisha Weller, Sean Hilton, 2006
Third edition text © Mark Levy, Sean Hilton, Greta Barnes 2000
Cartoons © Class Publishing

All rights reserved. Without limiting the rights under copyright reserved above, no part of this publication may be reproduced, stored in or introduced into a retrieval system, or transmitted, in any form or by any means (electronic, mechanical, photocopying, recording or otherwise), without the prior written permission of the publisher of this book.

The authors assert their rights as set out in Sections 77 and 78 of the Copyright Designs and Patents Act 1988 to be identified as the authors of this work wherever it is published commercially and whenever any adaptation of this work is published or produced including any sound recordings or files made of or based upon this work.

*Printing history*
First published 1993; Reprinted 1993, 1994; Revised edition 1994;
Reprinted 1996; Second edition 1997; Reprinted 1997; Third edition 2000;
Fourth edition 2006

The information presented in this book is accurate and current to the best of the authors' knowledge. The authors and publisher, however, make no guarantee as to, and assume no responsibility for, the correctness, sufficiency or completeness of such information or recommendation. The reader is advised to consult a doctor regarding all aspects of individual health care.

Products mentioned in the text are trademarks of the manufacturers listed in the Appendix.

The authors and publisher welcome feedback from the users of this book. Please contact the publisher.

**Class Publishing (London) Ltd,**
**Barb House, Barb Mews, London W6 7PA**
**Telephone: 020 7371 2119**
**Fax: 020 7371 2878 [International +4420]**
**Email: post@class.co.uk**
**Website: www.class.co.uk**

A CIP catalogue record for this book is available from the British Library

ISBN 10: 1 85959 111 6

ISBN 13: 978 1 85959 111 6

Edited by Michèle Clarke

Illustrations by David Woodroffe

Cartoons by Jenny Hartree (www.wildartworks.com)

Typeset by Martin Bristow

Printed and bound in Finland by WS Bookwell, Juva

# Contents

*Acknowledgements*     xiii

*Foreword by Professor Martyn Partridge MD, FRCP*     xv

INTRODUCTION

What this book is about and how to use it     1

How to beat your asthma     4

How to use this book     5

CHAPTER 1 *What is asthma and how does it affect people?*     7

Asthma explained     8

Types of asthma     12

About asthma     15

Inheritance     18

CHAPTER 2 *Symptoms and triggers of asthma*     23

Symptoms     24

Triggers     28

Related conditions     42

CHAPTER 3 *How is asthma diagnosed?*                          45
   When should asthma be suspected?                           47
   Diagnosis of asthma – tests and investigations            50
   Blowing tests: peak expiratory flow and spirometry        51
   Is it really asthma, and is there more than one type?     58
   What other diseases can be incorrectly diagnosed
      instead of asthma?                                     61

CHAPTER 4 *Treatments for Asthma*                             68
   Non-medicine treatments                                   69
   Medicines                                                 79

CHAPTER 5 *Beating asthma*                                   127
   Seeing the doctor, the asthma nurse – and asthma clinics  131
   Recognizing uncontrolled asthma – preventing attacks      140
   Peak expiratory flow monitoring                           145
   Written action plans for asthma                           157
   Altering and changing treatment                           162

CHAPTER 6 *Living with asthma*                               170
   Everyday life                                             172
   Smoking                                                   181
   Sex, periods, pregnancy and the menopause                 185
   Work                                                      193
   Holidays                                                  198
   Sport                                                     204
   Pollution and weather                                     209
   Food and drink                                            212
   Asthma and the National Health Service                    216
   The long-term outlook                                     219

CHAPTER 7 *Children and asthma*                      224
  How and when does asthma start?                   226
  Infants                                           231
  Childhood                                         234
  At school                                         240
  Growing out of it?                                244
  Adolescents and young adults                      246

CHAPTER 8 *Emergencies*                              249
  Symptoms and warnings                             251
  First aid for emergencies                         255

CHAPTER 9 *Self-help for asthma*                     273
  Asthma charities                                  274
  Information about asthma                           276

GLOSSARY                                             282

APPENDIX
  Useful addresses, information and websites        295

INDEX                                                303

# Dedication

*This book is for Celia, Lesley and Peter,
for all their helpful comments,
input and support.*

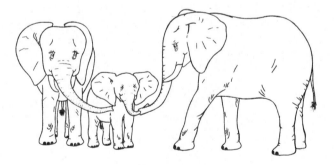

# Acknowledgements

We should like to thank all those asthma nurses who took the time to ask their patients for questions on asthma and we are indebted to those people with asthma who kindly provided us the genuine questions used in this book.

We should like to thank Education for Health (incorporating the National Respiratory Training Centre and Heartsave) for providing line illustrations of devices, and Asthma UK for permission to use illustrations of their leaflets.

Thanks are also due to Mrs Carol Bennett for her useful comments on the 3rd edition of this book, which helped us in the writing of the 4th edition.

The box in Chapter 9 is reproduced courtesy of the Royal College of Physicians, from *Clinical Effectiveness and Evaluation Unit: measuring clinical outcome in asthma*. London: RCP, 1999.

Finally, thanks to Jenny Hartree (www.wildartworks.com) for the elephant cartoons.

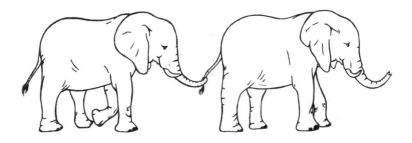

# Foreword

by Professor Martyn R. Partridge MD, FRCP

*Chief Medical Adviser, Asthma UK; Professor of
Respiratory Medicine, NHLI Division, Imperial College London,
and Consultant Chest Physician, Hammersmith Hospitals NHS Trust*

Most people with asthma will have only very limited contact with healthcare professionals during the average year. It is likely that for over 364 days the person with asthma, or the person who cares for the person with asthma, looks after their own condition. To do this satisfactorily necessitates the person with asthma having an understanding of the condition, knowing the purpose of their medications and being able to recognize when their asthma is worsening and what to do under those circumstances. Acquisition of that knowledge and those skills should be available from doctors and nurses but time within consultations is inevitably limited and we all forget some things which we have been told!

*Asthma – the 'at your fingertips' guide* is a unique resource for people with asthma and it provides the information necessary for them to take control of their condition.

In most countries of the world, the prevalence of asthma has increased dramatically over the last three decades. However, despite that, there are encouraging signs that the numbers who sadly die from this condition are falling and the numbers of people being admitted to hospital are also falling. This reflects the better medication which we have available but it's essential that all with this common condition benefit maximally from those therapies and feel comfortable taking them. We should be grateful to the authors of this book for providing us with such clear advice and information about asthma.

# Introduction

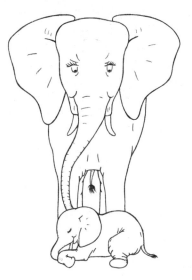

## *What this book is about and how to use it*

Asthma is one of the commonest long-term conditions and in the UK around 5 million people have it. In 2004 UK health professional asthma experts produced updated national guidelines for the management of asthma. They agreed that people with asthma need information and education about their condition. This should be aimed at individual needs and backed up with written asthma action plans. There are certain basic principles and skills that need to be understood, however mild the asthma is.

This book contains that basic information; it also has more detailed information for anyone with more complex asthma, or who may have had asthma for many years and wants to ask more 'advanced' questions. As in previous editions of our book, this 4th edition provides clear answers to 'real questions' from our patients. We have, however, changed the layout of the chapters to make it easier for you to learn more about your asthma.

We answer real, practical questions of importance for anyone interested in asthma and we help people with asthma and their families to understand more about their condition. In this way, we aim to help anyone with asthma live life to the full. It is essential that people and families understand how to recognize worsening asthma and avoid asthma attacks. If you have asthma or are a relative or close friend of someone who has, we know you will find the book helpful. We believe that it is vital for you to be involved in your own care (that is in 'self-care' or 'self-management') as you are the person who lives with asthma day in and day out. In this book we shall provide you with information and practical tips that enable you to manage your asthma and reduce the problems it can cause you.

In the first chapters, we help you to understand how variable asthma is and how it affects people. We also explain the things that make asthma worse, so you can try to avoid them. We believe it is important to have a basic understanding of respiratory signs and symptoms and how asthma is diagnosed – this is covered in Chapter 3 *How is asthma diagnosed?* It is helpful to recognize when you need to worry about asthma, because these same signs and symptoms also occur when asthma goes out of control. This will help you to know when to take extra asthma medicines or to call for help.

For the sections covering asthma medicines, we have tried to be consistent in the names we have used. There are many brand names for anti-asthma medicines, as well as the true (or generic) names, and we realize that these can be confusing. Where a particular name has been included in the question we have continued to use that name. You will find more detail about the different medicines and inhaler devices used for asthma in Chapter 4 *Treatments for asthma.*

Throughout the book you will find frequent references to peak flow meters and peak expiratory flow (PEF) readings. The peak flow meter is a small and simple piece of equipment that measures how hard you can blow (see Figure 5.1 in Chapter 5). When your *airways* are narrowed, such as during an asthma attack, the reading you get on the meter scale will be reduced. When you are well, the reading will be higher. We believe that monitoring the peak expiratory flow, combined with recognizing the presence of asthma symptoms, is the best way to keep a check on your asthma (rather like using a blood pressure machine to measure blood pressure). This does not mean that we believe everyone with asthma should be using peak flow meters all the time, but when problems arise they do give the best assessment of how severe the asthma is. There is a section in Chapter 5 ***Beating asthma*** on the use of peak flow meters.

Unfortunately there is no cure for asthma at the present time, but for most people it is possible to keep their symptoms under excellent control. With a good understanding of asthma, you should be able to recognize the danger signs of when it is out of control, and information in this book will help you to learn how to recognize and treat these episodes. Many people are troubled unnecessarily by their asthma because they are not receiving the right treatment, or because they do not realize the benefits of current asthma treatments. Sections in Chapters 5, 6 and 8 provide information on self-management and what to do in asthma emergencies.

Chapter 7 ***Children and asthma*** provides information that is of importance for parents, but we hope that they will find the rest of the book valuable as well.

Inevitably, some of the terms we use are medical or technical. We have tried to explain these terms wherever they occur, and have attempted to steer clear of medical jargon. We have also included a glossary of some of the more important (and perhaps confusing) medical terms that tend to come up time and time again. When these terms are first mentioned in the book, we have italicised them, e.g. *bronchial hyperreactivity*.

## *How to beat your asthma*

The major challenge is to find ways of living with asthma without the illness interfering too much with daily life. In this book, we support a problem-solving approach, first by making sure that you get the information you need on asthma. This will help you to live with asthma. For some people, having asthma is a problem and people solve problems in different ways. Problem solving has several stages:

- It begins with identifying or clarifying a particular problem (for example, your asthma is making you breathless when you run), and then trying to imagine where you want to be in the future (for example, to be able to run without getting breathless).

- The next stage is to try to figure out how you are going to get from where you are to where you want to be. Gathering this information allows you to find out as much as you can about the cause of the problem and how to fix it.

- Next you see how this information applies to you (for example, you might want to prove that your asthma is indeed the cause of your breathlessness, perhaps by using a peak flow meter).

- Finally you then find ways of using this information to solve the problem (for example, agreeing an asthma action plan with your doctor or asthma nurse).

Each chapter starts with a number of learning points so that you can focus your thoughts on these while reading the chapter. We suggest that, as you read through the book, you think about questions that are important for you, and write them down. You may wish to ask your doctor or asthma nurse about these questions when you next go to the surgery. We have tried to help by ending each chapter with a number of suggested questions. In this way, we hope to give you a structured approach to finding out about asthma and using what you learn, to help you live a life unrestricted by asthma.

# *How to use this book*

Because people have differing needs for information about asthma, this book has been designed in a way that means you do not have to read it from cover to cover. The questions are arranged into chapters and sections; you may want to dip into sections, or look for the answer to a particular question you have on your asthma, by using the contents table and the index.

- If you have just been diagnosed as having asthma, we suggest that you concentrate on the following sections first:
- *What is asthma?* (Chapter 1)
- *Symptoms* and *Triggers* in Chapter 2
- *Medicines* in Chapter 4
- *Emergencies* (Chapter 8).

If you are more experienced in managing your own asthma, you may wish to concentrate more on the peak expiratory flow rate sections in Chapters 3 and 5.

If your child has asthma, we hope that Chapter 7 will deal with many of your concerns.

This style means that inevitably there will be some repetition within the book, and a few questions will appear to be duplicated in different sections. There is some cross-referencing of questions, but we have tried to keep this to a minimum. We prefer to answer each question in full, rather than direct you to a number of different sections each time, but for reasons of space this is not always possible.

This book has been written from *real* questions that we have been asked by hundreds of *real* people with *real* asthma! Not everyone will agree that the questions we have chosen are the important ones, and certainly not everyone will agree with the answers we have provided. Each edition of this book has been improved by feedback from the people who know most about problems relating to asthma – you! We really hope that you will enjoy this book and find it helpful in controlling your asthma.

If you have any comments about the contents of this book we will be delighted to receive them. Please write to us, c/o Class Publishing, Barb House, Barb Mews, London W6 7PA, UK.

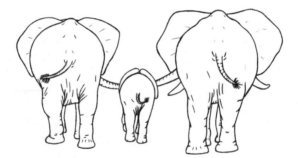

# 1
# What is asthma and how does it affect people?

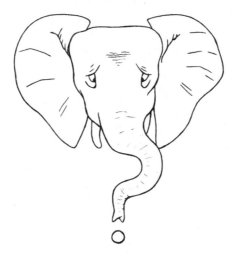

**In this chapter you will learn about:**

- what asthma is

- what happens to the airways if you have asthma

- why people with asthma sometimes die from a bad asthma attack

- the 'hygiene hypothesis' (a possible explanation for the increase in asthma in recent years)

- the likelihood of inheriting asthma.

In the UK there are around 5 million people with asthma. Asthma is the commonest chronic condition affecting children, with 1 in 7 of all children having asthma at any one time.

Asthma varies in severity both in adults and in children. It may be mild, with only an occasional need for treatment, but a small proportion of people have very severe asthma, with repeated admissions to hospital, and a restricted lifestyle. Fortunately the great majority of people with asthma are able to lead a full life, either free from symptoms or with minimal symptoms. Nevertheless, few health conditions have a greater impact than asthma. It is estimated that the annual cost of asthma care in the UK is over 2 billion pounds. These costs are related to health care provided by the National Health Service, social security payments in the form of invalidity payments from the Department of Social Security, and lost productivity, as a result of sickness and absence from work.

When you are first told that you have asthma, many thoughts will flash through your mind. If you have a close friend or relative with asthma, you will wonder whether your own asthma will be like theirs. No two people have the same pattern of symptoms, and even for the same person, symptoms can vary in severity at different times. The important points to learn are:

- about your own asthma
- how it affects you
- what makes it worse, and
- how your treatment can help.

Do not be overinfluenced by what happens to other people – we are all different!

## *Asthma explained*

**What is asthma?**

We have two *lungs*, which are often described as being like a pair of large sponges (see Figure 1.1). They are situated in our chest and are essential for breathing oxygen into our bloodstream and breathing carbon dioxide out.

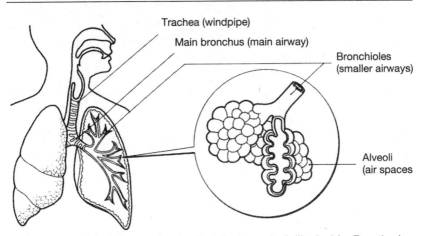

**Figure 1.1** This diagram shows what the lungs look like inside. Breathed air goes from the windpipe (trachea) into the two main airways (bronchi). From there it goes through the small bronchioles to the air spaces (alveoli) and then is absorbed into the bloodstream.

Asthma is a condition that causes occasional tightening of the air passages, which makes it difficult breathing air in and out of the lungs. This occasional or varying tightening is characteristic of asthma. Most people are fit and well in between attacks or episodes, and can breathe normally.

It might be easier to appreciate the structure of the lungs if they are likened to an upside-down tree. Here, the tree trunk is similar to the main windpipe, or *trachea*; the larger branches are the main airways (main *bronchi*). The smaller branches resemble the smaller airways (bronchi) and the twigs represent the very small airways (*bronchioles*). The air sacs or *alveoli* are represented by the leaves.

Air is breathed in through the nose and mouth and into the main windpipe, or trachea. Air then travels though the larger branches (the main bronchus) and to smaller branches (the bronchi) and then to even smaller airways, or bronchioles. At the end of the air passages the air reaches the air sacs, or alveoli. It is in the air sacs that oxygen passes from the air into the bloodstream and the waste product, carbon dioxide, is passed in the opposite direction, out of the blood into the air sacs. This is known as gas exchange or 'respiration'. If you have asthma, this affects your bronchi. They

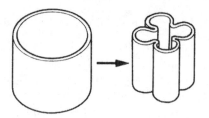

**a** Tightening of airways from muscle spasm with reduced space

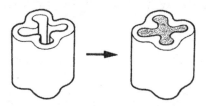

**b** Swelling of walls, with production of thick mucus

**Figure 1.2** In asthma the airways narrow owing to spasm (tightening) of the muscles around them and swelling of the lining and sticky mucus inside them.

become narrow, which makes it more difficult for air to move to and from the air sacs (see Figure 1.2). Asthma is sometimes referred to as bronchial asthma.

### Is cardiac asthma the same as bronchial asthma?

*Cardiac asthma* and bronchial asthma both cause difficulty in breathing, but for different reasons. Cardiac asthma is an old-fashioned term used to describe acute heart failure (the term 'cardiac' refers to the heart). In heart failure, the heart muscle is not able to pump blood around the body efficiently and the lungs become filled with fluid, causing breathing problems. In cardiac asthma, the air sacs are filled with fluid, whereas in bronchial asthma air has difficulty in reaching the air sacs because the breathing tubes are narrowed.

**Is asthma caused by the airways becoming narrower?**

Asthma symptoms are the result of airways becoming narrower, and as a result it is more difficult for air to get in and out of the lungs (see Figure 1.2). The symptoms of asthma are wheezing, coughing and shortness of breath. Although the airways become narrow, the underlying problem is *inflammation* of the lining of the airways. The exact cause of asthma is often unknown, but there are many things that can irritate the airways and lead to the inflammation.

**My asthma nurse says my airways are inflamed. What does this mean?**

Tightness in the airways leads to narrowing and the lining of these airways can become sore and swollen; this is known as inflammation. Airways become inflamed in response to something that irritates them. The lining of the airways become swollen, and small glands in this lining produce lots of sticky mucus or phlegm. Inflammation of the airways causes coughing, as does the tightening of the muscles that surround the airways. The inflamed airways are sometimes referred to as *twitchy airways* because they are very sensitive and irritable.

As a result of inflammation, the airway size, or diameter, is reduced in three ways:

- tightness or spasm of the muscles around the airways (Figure 1.2a)
- swelling of the airway lining (Figure 1.2b)
- production of sticky mucus which tends to block it (Figure 1.2b).

**Is asthma a virus?**

Asthma is not a *virus*. A virus is a germ that causes illness of all sorts, from the common cold and measles, to hepatitis, influenza, cold sores and many, many other conditions. There are thousands of different types of viruses. Virus infections do not get better with antibiotic medicines.

There is, however, an important link between asthma and viruses. The link is that the most common *trigger* of an attack or episode of asthma is an *upper respiratory tract infection* (common cold) – caused by a virus. A type of virus known as the *rhinovirus* is often responsible, but there are others, including the influenza virus. This is why it is important for people with asthma to be immunized against the 'flu. If you have a cold that 'goes to your chest' and makes your asthma worse, remember that it is likely to be a virus infection responsible for it.

# Types of asthma

### Is my asthma an allergy?

Asthma and *allergy* are not the same thing but they often go together. If you have an allergy, it means that you have an oversensitive response to things that most people do not react to. If you are allergic to something that you breathe in, it can cause symptoms of wheezing, itchy eyes or a runny nose. The substances that trigger an *allergic reaction* are known as *allergens*. An allergic reaction does not happen the first time you come into contact with a particular allergen. It usually develops over a period of time after repeat or subsequent exposure to the allergen.

Grass pollen, *house dust mite* and pet hair are some of the everyday things that can cause an allergic reaction in some people. Asthma is often triggered by an allergic reaction and, if you are allergic to cats, just handling, stroking, or even being in the same room as one can produce symptoms.

Sometimes it is easy to identify the allergen that triggers asthma symptoms; at other times it is very difficult. Once the allergen has been identified, avoiding or reducing the amount of contact with that asthma trigger is sensible but it is not always easy to do so.

**My doctor talks about different types of asthma. What does this mean?**

There are different types of asthma that may or may not be a result of an allergic response. Asthma can be triggered by:

- allergy

- infection

- hormone changes

- an irritant

- environmental factors.

Asthma commonly starts in childhood (often referred to as '*early-onset asthma*') or it may start in adult life (known as '*late-onset asthma*'). In addition people may develop asthma symptoms for various reasons:

- as a result of exercise

- only in the *hay fever* (pollen) season (sometimes called 'pollen asthma')

- because of their work environment (this is called *occupational asthma* if it starts for the first time at work; if asthma has been made worse by exposure to substances at work it is known as 'work-aggravated asthma').

Exercise symptoms are a common asthma trigger, and there are some people who only ever have asthma symptoms following some sort of exercise. If exercise is infrequent, then a reliever inhaler medicine immediately beforehand is likely to be the only treatment required. If someone does a lot of exercise, then asthma symptoms will be more frequent, and likely to be more of a nuisance. In this situation, a *preventer* and a *reliever* asthma inhaler will control asthma symptoms better than just a reliever.

Pollen asthma, as the name suggests, happens in the pollen or 'hay fever' season. The pollen season lasts from February right through to September, but there are three distinct phases:

- early or late spring as a result of tree pollens
- in June or July as a result of grass pollens
- in July to September as a result of mould spores.

Although pollen is a common asthma trigger, few people are unlucky enough to be troubled through all three phases of the pollen season.

If asthma symptoms do not happen at any other time of the year, asthma treatment can be started a few weeks before the known pollen trigger and continued for as long as it is around.

Asthma varies greatly in how severe it is; when mild and infrequent it is referred to as episodic or occasional. At other times asthma may be persistent (*chronic*) or persistent (chronic) severe. Mild or episodic asthma is usually triggered by the common cold.

**I have no relatives with asthma, and now at the age of 42 I have developed asthma. Why me?**

Asthma is very common and about 1 in 20 (5%) of adults develop it. It may develop at any age and sometimes there is no inherited factor. Just as asthma can be triggered by a virus infection (such as a cold) in young children, it can also be triggered by a respiratory infection later in life. It is possible that this is what has happened to you, but it is also possible that your asthma is due to occupational exposure. If you are working in one of the occupations that are associated with asthma, you should ask your doctor or asthma nurse to check for this (see the question **What is occupational asthma?** in Chapter 6).

If you had asthma as a child, it is possible that it has returned. Childhood asthma is sometimes undiagnosed especially if the respiratory symptoms are mild. The symptoms are often referred to as '*bronchitis*' or 'chestiness'. These respiratory symptoms tend to improve and settle down later in childhood but for some reason recur later on in adult life; this might have happened with you.

Throughout this book we emphasize that the severity of asthma varies enormously. Many people feel very worried and depressed when they are told that they have asthma; others feel disbelief or are angry. However, once they know more about their asthma and the fact that it can be treated successfully, most find that these feelings go away and they come to terms with their condition.

Having asthma can still carry an unnecessary stigma and some people feel ashamed and wish to avoid anyone knowing about it. This is a pity (and wrong!) but it could well date from the time when asthma was wrongly thought to be psychological in origin. 'Nervous' asthma was thought to be the fault of the patient, not the environment or their genes. If you have asthma, it is nobody's fault. Fortunately, modern asthma treatments help you to be free from symptoms at all times and able to lead a full life with no restrictions on what you can do, rather than feeling stigmatized or different.

## *About asthma*

### Is asthma catching? Can I give it to my children?

You cannot catch asthma because it is not an infectious disease, but there are reasons why some people think this is the case because:

- you *can* catch a cold, which may make asthma worse
- asthma often runs in families and some people believe that it is an infectious disease
- asthma is more common now and people believe (wrongly) that the disease is 'spreading' like an infectious disease.

### How did my asthma start – and why?

Without knowing all the details of your *medical history*, we cannot say how or why you have asthma, but we can give you some idea about what is currently known about the causes of asthma.

We have already mentioned that the airways become twitchy and irritable. The medical term for this twitchiness is *bronchial hyperreactivity* (BHR). This simply means that the bronchi overreact. In children it may be a single virus infection (such as a cold) or frequent respiratory infections that make the airways twitchy and irritable. Coming into contact with substances early in life, to which we might be allergic (such as pets or high house dust mite levels), may switch on BHR and lead to childhood asthma.

Usually the tendency to develop asthma is inherited. This is called a 'genetic predisposition' and is described in more detail in the section on *Inheritance* in this chapter. However, as with many other conditions, it is a combination of genetic and environmental factors that actually leads to the appearance of asthma and the actual symptoms.

There is increasing evidence that the environment in which we live plays an important role in the development of allergy. We now know that mothers who smoke during pregnancy have babies who are more likely to develop allergic antibodies. Antibodies are substances that are produced by our *immune system* and are part of our own defence mechanisms, but allergic antibodies may be harmful and lead to the appearance of allergy.

### Can asthma be cured?

No, asthma cannot be cured but it can be controlled by effective treatment. Asthma symptoms may disappear with effective treatment, and may sometimes disappear even without treatment. Asthma is therefore called a variable condition. There are times when people feel that they must be cured because they are completely without symptoms. While this symptomless state (called *remission*) can go on for a long time, once you have had asthma you will always have the potential to have it again, even years later. It is probably better to think of asthma going into remission rather than being cured.

### I read in the local paper that someone had died as a result of an asthma attack. Why does this happen?

It is always tragic when someone dies from asthma, particularly as many asthma deaths are preventable. Fortunately, such deaths are relatively rare, but in the UK there are still about 1400 people who die from severe asthma attacks each year. Because asthma is so common and usually mild, it is easy to think 'it's only asthma', but it is important to remember that asthma can have very serious consequences. Taking regular preventer asthma treatment will help to control asthma, but all too often people do not take their preventer inhaler medicines. This is for a whole variety of reasons including:

- forgetting to take their asthma treatment
- not recognizing how serious their asthma attack is
- not having the right amount of asthma treatment
- having other things or problems in their life that are more important than their asthma treatment
- not believing they have asthma
- not wanting to take a 'medicine' regularly.

A small number of people have very severe and unstable asthma despite taking their asthma medicines. This is called *brittle asthma* or chronic severe asthma. Occasionally some deaths do occur in this group because of the seriousness of the asthma.

### Do children die from asthma?

Yes they do, but fortunately asthma deaths in children are extremely rare. Fewer than 50 of the 1400 or so deaths per year in the UK occur in children under the age of 16, but it is heart-rending when a child dies from a treatable disease. The reasons include those listed in the previous question. In childhood, the parents' knowledge, beliefs and commitment to asthma treatment are as equally important as the child's own reaction to asthma.

Very rarely, children do die as a result of their first asthma attack. They may have had very minor asthma symptoms in the past, which may have been ignored or not thought of as serious. It is worth remembering that children with severe food allergy (e.g. nut allergy) are at risk of dying from asthma during an allergic attack. Fortunately such deaths are extremely rare but for many parents this often leaves them with the unanswered question: 'Could I have done something to prevent my child's death?'

# Inheritance

### Why have I got asthma?

There is not always a clear answer to this reasonable question! People may feel singled out because they have asthma, but others almost expect it because it runs so strongly in their families. We know that some of our characteristics (like the colour of our eyes) and some rare diseases (such as haemophilia) can be caused by inheriting single *genes* but it is likely that a number of different genes play a role in the asthma tendency (see the next question). Genes are important because they give us our own unique identification.

Viral infections of the respiratory system (e.g. colds) usually set off changes in the linings of the airways, leading to asthma symptoms; for others allergies are the trigger. Adults in certain occupations may also develop asthma as a result of substances they come into contact with at work.

Some people with an inherited tendency to develop asthma may go through their entire lives and not develop it, despite encountering these trigger factors many times. This is just one more mystery showing how much we still don't understand about the cause of asthma.

### I read that the asthma gene has been discovered. Can I expect a cure for my asthma now?

You are right – an important asthma gene has been discovered, which is really exciting, but it is likely to be many years before we can begin to talk of cures. This asthma gene is called Adam 33 and was discovered in recent years. There are dedicated researchers involved with this exciting discovery and they are continuing their research in this area trying to understand how this particular gene interacts with others.

**People say that we have more asthma now because we are too clean and hygienic. Is that true?**

The UK has one of the highest levels of asthma in the world. In the developed world there is certainly much more asthma than in the developing world. How we acquire the asthma tendency is not fully understood, but there are some suggestions that changes in our body's defence system (immune system) are partly responsible for this, because we are not exposed to infections early in life. This suggestion or theory is called the 'hygiene hypothesis' but it has not been proven conclusively. Another possible factor contributing to this theory is that family sizes are smaller, with fewer opportunities for common infections to be passed on to young babies from older brothers and sisters.

Babies are born with their immune system having a tendency towards an allergic response. According to the hygiene hypothesis, if you are exposed to lots of infections early in life, these infections are thought to 'switch off' the allergic tendency of the immune system. Less developed countries do not have as much asthma as the 'western' world, possibly because the levels of hygiene are not as good and parasite infections are more common. In the western world we are very conscious of sterilizing and making sure everything is ultra-clean for our babies. This means that they are not exposed to the everyday germs and their immune system does not have to cope with potential infections.

**As asthma runs in families is there anything I can do to prevent my children from getting it?**

There is some evidence to suggest that children who are exposed to allergy-causing substances in the first few months of life are more likely to develop asthma later in childhood, particularly where there is a history of allergy in the family.

Babies born between March and May are exposed to high pollen levels and those born in the early winter months arrive when the house dust mite is at its most active. So if you want to try to reduce the chances of your child developing an allergic condition (asthma, hay fever or *eczema*), then you need to plan the birth for between December and February!

There is confusing information about breastfeeding and whether it protects your baby against asthma or other atopic (allergic) conditions such as eczema. Looking at the different scientific information, the conclusion is that breastfeeding does not **definitely** prevent the development of allergic diseases. However, breastfeeding does give a baby the best possible start in life by providing them with the perfect milk formula and should be encouraged whenever possible.

### Can the development of asthma be halted by avoiding important allergens during pregnancy and in early infancy?

Research so far links parents who smoke (particularly mothers) with increased numbers of children with respiratory illnesses. All parents of young children should be advised not to smoke, but even more so if they or their relatives have asthma, hay fever or allergies. Avoiding smoking completely is worthwhile because it is known that smoking in pregnancy and during the early months of a baby's life increases allergy antibodies (substances produced by the immune system).

### I already have one child with asthma. If I have other children, is it likely that they will have it too?

Yes, it is. You have a much greater chance of having a child with asthma if you or any of your close relatives already have asthma. It is also more likely if you or the child's father is *atopic*. Being atopic, means that you have a tendency to develop one or more of the following conditions: asthma, eczema or hay fever. If you and your partner are both atopic, then your baby will have about a 1 in 2 chance of developing an atopic condition – but, of course, this may not be asthma. (See also question on atopy in Chapter 3.)

Studies carried out on the families of infants with asthma suggest that there is an inherited (or genetic) element, which influences the development of what is known as bronchial hyperreactivity (or 'twitchy airways'). This inherited element probably has an effect only if something in the environment influences it and 'switches' it on.

There are other things that may be associated with asthma, and that may affect your children. Bottle-fed babies are more likely to develop allergic problems (and therefore asthma) than those who are breastfed for more than 3 months. Children in small families and from more wealthy homes are also more likely to develop allergic conditions. Children from families who smoke have more chest problems, including asthma.

### I have had asthma since childhood. Will my children have asthma?

There is no doubt that all atopic (allergic) conditions, such as asthma, hay fever and eczema, run in families. If both parents are atopic, there is a greater chance of having a child with asthma, or either of the other atopic conditions for that matter, than if they are non-atopic.

### I'm over 60 and have just been diagnosed as having asthma. I've never had any problem before – why have I got asthma now?

Asthma can occur at any time of life. It can start for the first time in a premature baby or in someone in their later years (late-onset asthma). What we can't tell you is why you have developed asthma now. One of the commonest reasons for people to develop asthma for the first time between the ages of 40 and 60 years – or beyond, as in your case – is as a result of a severe episode of 'bronchitis', or a chest infection. They may seem to make a slow but full recovery, only for their chesty symptoms to return. The coughing, wheezing and breathlessness can be very distressing, and these chesty symptoms are often worse at night.

You haven't said whether you are a man or a woman, but we know that, in your age group, more women than men develop asthma. Unfortunately many adults who develop asthma are wrongly diagnosed as having bronchitis, even if they have never smoked or lived and worked in a polluted environment. If bronchitis is diagnosed, this often means that the doctor does not prescribe anti-asthma medicines. It is good that your condition has been diagnosed, because it means that you should receive the correct asthma medicines.

---

**Personal action plan – things you might wish to discuss with your doctor or asthma nurse**

If you or your child has been recently diagnosed with asthma, you will benefit from having a personal action plan (self-management plan). This will help you to recognize asthma attacks and know what to do when they occur. When you visit your doctor or asthma nurse, you might like to make a note of any of the points below in order to discuss them further during the consultation. Do ask your doctor or asthma nurse for more information on asthma and asthma action plans.

- If you are an adult with newly diagnosed asthma, is this due to your occupation?

- What are the trigger factors that make your asthma worse?

- Which medication should you take, and when?

- If you are planning to have children, how can you minimize the likelihood of them developing asthma?

---

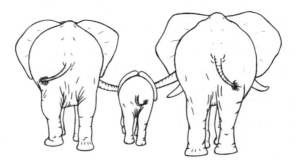

# 2
# Symptoms and triggers of asthma

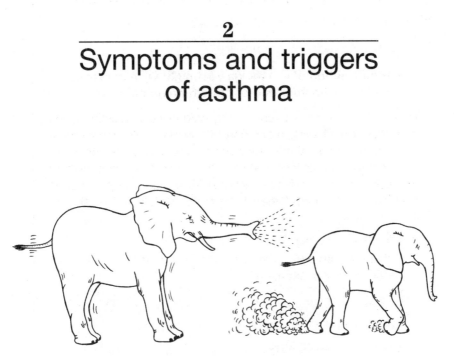

In this chapter you will learn about:

- asthma symptoms

- how asthma symptoms make your asthma worse

- asthma triggers

- how asthma triggers make your asthma worse

- other conditions that may have an effect on your asthma.

# Symptoms

**What are the symptoms of asthma?**

The main symptoms of asthma are:

- **Coughing**. When the airways are irritable and sensitive (twitchy), this irritation can make you cough. The coughing is often worse at night.

- **Wheezing**. When the airways in the lungs become tight, they narrow in size. This makes it more difficult to breathe out normally and air has to be forced out instead. If air is forced out of the lungs through narrowed airways, it causes a high pitched squeaky or whistling noise known as wheezing.

- **Chest tightness**. When the airways become narrow, it can give you the feeling that there is something tight around the chest, and this makes breathing uncomfortable. It can be quite painful too and, because of this, you may think something is wrong with your heart, but asthma does not affect the heart in this way.

- **Shortness of breath**. When the airways are tight, breathing is harder than normal and results in shortness of breath, especially on exertion.

**Why is my asthma worse at night?**

Nobody knows the answer to this question for sure. It is fair to say that most things seem to be worse at night – from toothache to anxiety.

We do know that, when we are asleep, the airways are more relaxed and they become slightly floppy. That means that there is less air going in and out of the lungs as we breathe. We know this because, if you do peak flow blowing tests first thing in the morning, you will find that the readings are slightly lower than they are in the evening. This is quite normal and happens even if you do not have asthma. As well as the airways becoming relaxed at night, some of the 'body rhythm' hormones that our body produces are lower and so we function more slowly.

If your asthma is not under control, asthma symptoms of coughing or wheezing are worse at night and can wake you up. They may disturb others in your family too, even if they do not disturb you! Talk to your asthma nurse or doctor about any night-time asthma symptoms because they may be able to suggest treatment changes that will help to get your asthma under better control.

### Why does my chest feel tight?

Wheezing is only one of the symptoms of asthma and we know that some people hardly ever wheeze. The other main symptoms are coughing and shortness of breath. Chest tightness, such as you describe, is another common symptom. Asthma causes narrowing of the airways in three ways:

- mucus (phlegm) inside the airways

- thickening (swelling) of the walls of the airways

- muscle contraction (tightening) in the walls of the airways. (See Figure 1.2 in the previous chapter.)

This narrowing of the airways causes wheezing, but some people report little or no wheezing if airway narrowing is minimal. In mild asthma there is often just a persistent dry cough, or some shortness of breath on exertion.

### When I had a bad asthma attack my doctor said he couldn't hear any wheezing. What did he mean by that?

There is an entirely different occasion in asthma where no wheeze may be heard at all. During a bad asthma attack (also known as an *acute* severe asthma attack), if your airways are very tight, it is very difficult for air to get into or out of your lungs. This means that the wheezing noise of air forcing its way through narrow airway tubes cannot be heard when your doctor or asthma nurse listens to your chest with a stethoscope. In a bad asthma attack this lack of wheezing is known as a *silent chest*. If this occurs, the person having the bad asthma attack may look blue (you can see that their lips or tongue are blue), because it means that their blood does not have enough oxygen. This is a life-threatening situation and urgent medical help is needed. Phone the emergency services (dial 999 in the UK) immediately for help and tell them the person is having a severe asthma attack.

**As asthma is a lung condition, why is it that my throat seems to close so that I feel as if I'm being strangled?**

Your lungs contain thousands of air passages, which range in size from the main windpipe (trachea) starting in the throat to the smallest airways, the bronchioles, which empty into the air spaces, the alveoli (see Figure 1.1 in the previous chapter). Asthma affects all of these air passages to some degree. In the majority of people it is the smaller air passages deep inside the lungs that are most affected. However, in some people – like you – it affects mainly the larger ones, even up to the trachea, and this is why you have a sensation of being strangled during an attack. Not only is this very unpleasant for you, but it tends to be slower to respond to treatment than the more common form.

**Can I get rid of my asthma symptoms?**

It is not possible to get rid of your asthma but it is certainly possible to get rid of your symptoms so that your asthma is under control: this is what you and your asthma doctor or nurse should aim for. If you are having continuing symptoms, your doctor will review and reassess your asthma medicines. Symptoms are not 'normal' or 'to be expected' but are a sign of incomplete asthma control. It is essential not only to be prescribed the right treatment, but also to take it regularly! You must be able to use your inhaler device correctly too! Your asthma nurse or doctor can check this when you attend for an asthma review. Your pharmacist may also be able to help.

**My son experienced a rash while suffering an asthmatic cough. Is this rare and are the two connected?**

People do occasionally complain of itching when they have a flare-up of their asthma. However, we are not aware of any relationship between an asthma cough and a rash. There may be several explanations, but one of the commonest complications of any treatment with medicines is a skin rash. Exact figures are difficult to obtain, but it is known that about 3 in every 100 people who take medicines will develop a medicine-related rash. If your son was taking a different treatment for his cough at the time the rash developed, then this could be the cause, rather than his asthma. Some chest infections are also known to cause a temporary rash as well as make the asthma worse. This is particularly true of viral chest infections (similar to the common cold) in children.

Another possibility is that your son has atopic eczema. This is a skin inflammation that occurs in people who have an inherited tendency towards allergic problems. It often co-exists with other allergic conditions, especially asthma and hay fever. It is not uncommon for eczema to flare up at the same time as an episode of asthma.

**What causes the chest pain I get when my asthma is bad?**

There are three main causes of chest pain during uncontrolled asthma. These all occur as a result of stretching in the chest and any or all of them may be the cause of your pain.

- During an asthma attack the lungs expand greatly, because a lot of air becomes trapped in them. The *pleura* (which are membranes surrounding the lungs) stretch as a result, and this may cause pain.

- The walls of the chest stretch due to the overexpansion of the lungs. This causes strain on the rib joints (where the ribs join the breastbone, and at the back where they join the spine). This can also cause pain.

- The muscles between the ribs are stretched when the lungs are overexpanded, and this may be a third cause of the pain.

Many people immediately worry about a heart attack when chest pain is mentioned. Chest pain during asthma episodes rarely comes from the heart, unless it occurs in those people with known heart disease.

### Why do I have so little energy when my asthma is bad?

There may be a few reasons for this. When your asthma is bad and your airways become narrow, oxygen cannot get through them efficiently and this leads to a lack of energy. The main work of the lungs is to enable oxygen to get from the air to the blood (they also help to remove waste products like carbon dioxide from the body). Oxygen is essential for all the organs and tissues of the body, such as the heart, brain and kidneys. When the body is short of oxygen, these vital organs get tired and you feel short of energy. A virus infection is the commonest trigger for asthma and the virus itself often makes people feel tired.

# *Triggers*

### I have been told that I have an allergy, which is making my asthma worse. What does this mean?

Asthma is triggered by many things. For many people an allergy is the most important trigger of asthma symptoms or an asthma attack. The substance causing the allergy is known as an allergen, and it sets off an allergic reaction, which results in asthma symptoms. In the UK and much of the world, the house dust mite is the most important allergen to trigger asthma. These are tiny animals, related to spiders and ticks, which inhabit our homes in millions, living on scales of dead human skin. They are not visible to the human eye, but live in house dust, particularly in warm and moist conditions. Other important asthma allergic triggers include: feathers; animal fur or hair (known as animal *dander*) especially from cats, dogs and horses; grass and tree pollens, and mould spores.

Allergic *rhinitis* occurs when an allergen triggers nose symptoms: a runny, itchy or blocked nose. It is sometimes described as 'asthma of the nose' because there are many similarities between asthma and rhinitis. One type of allergic rhinitis, seasonal rhinitis, is an allergy to pollen; this is usually called hay fever. People with seasonal rhinitis usually find their asthma gets worse when the pollen count is high. In fact, people who have both allergic rhinitis and asthma tend to have more problems with their asthma; so it is important to take the medicines as discussed with your health professional, if you have both of these conditions. Treatment of the pollen allergy can help to prevent and control episodes of worsening asthma.

Another important type of allergy is one that can occur as a result of sensitivity to a substance in the work environment. This can lead to occupational asthma or asthma that is made worse at work (also known as work-aggravated asthma). (See the question **What is occupational asthma?** in Chapter 6.)

### What is an asthma trigger?

An asthma trigger is something that makes your asthma worse. There are lots of different things that can do this and an asthma trigger is not always an allergic reaction. The following are well-known triggers of asthma:

- upper respiratory tract viral infections (colds)
- environmental triggers, e.g. smoking, traffic fumes
- occupational triggers, e.g. flour, solder, latex
- emotional reactions, e.g. stress, laughter, excitement
- allergic triggers, e.g. animals (especially cats and dogs), house dust mite, birds, pollen
- hormones regulating the menstrual cycle and pregnancy.

### Do asthma triggers cause asthma?

Generally speaking asthma triggers do not cause asthma – they bring on asthma symptoms or attacks. Occupational triggers are perhaps the one type that can be thought of as actually causing asthma. The question on occupational triggers later on will give you more information about it. (See the question **What is occupational asthma?** in Chapter 6.)

### My son is 6 years old and has asthma. Why does a cold always go to his chest?

Most people with asthma will be familiar with the cold that 'goes to the chest'. Colds are more common in the autumn and winter time and they are caused by virus infections that affect the upper respiratory airway system (i.e. nose and throat). This stays as a 'head cold' for many people, but others, especially those with asthma, find that they quite rapidly develop chesty symptoms. In children, especially young children, colds are the commonest trigger for making asthma worse.

### I developed asthma when I was 45 years old. What do you think is the likely cause of it as no one in my family has ever had asthma before?

Some people develop asthma later in life, just as you have done. We are not really sure why this happens but sometimes a heavy cold 'goes to your chest' and can be the initial trigger of asthma. It is not an allergic reaction, but something that leads to the tendency for colds to trigger asthma symptoms. This is thought to happen because of the way the airway cells respond. You may find that, each time you have a cold, it goes to your chest quite quickly. The other cause of 'late-onset asthma' is occupational asthma. If you are working in an industry known to be associated with risks of developing occupational asthma you should consult your doctor or asthma nurse for tests.

Occupational asthma is sometimes the cause of late-onset asthma. There are a number of industries where there is increased risk of developing occupational asthma. This may start with rhinitis (runny, itchy nose with sneezing), which starts after beginning a new job. There is more about occupational asthma in Chapter 5.

It is worth remembering that the aim of modern asthma

management is for you to be free from symptoms at all times and to be able to lead a full life with no restrictions.

**Whenever I go upstairs I get wheezy and I am out of breath. Why?**

Some people do find that their symptoms get worse when they do anything that means an increase in their normal activity, such as climbing a flight of stairs. Usually, exertion or exercise takes a few minutes to bring on asthma symptoms. If you are struggling when you are just doing your usual daily activities, this is a sign that your asthma is not under control. You need to review your symptoms and treatments with your asthma nurse or doctor, because exercise symptoms can usually be controlled very effectively.

**My daughter is 4 years old. When she went to a birthday party recently, she got really excited and became very wheezy. Why was this?**

The thought of going to a party does tend to make young children get very excited. For a young child with asthma, excitement as well as laughter can bring on asthma symptoms. These symptoms can be treated with asthma inhaler medicines that relax and 'open up' the airways. If these wheezing episodes are happening frequently, your daughter should be reviewed by an asthma nurse or doctor. She may need a change in her asthma medicines.

If this wheezing has happened for the first time, do make an appointment for your daughter to see an asthma nurse or doctor to see whether she needs regular anti-asthma treatment.

**My teenage daughter has asthma, which is always worse when she is stressed. Why?**

Stress is caused by an emotional response to a situation. Emotional responses like stress, laughter and excitement can make asthma symptoms worse and even bring on an asthma attack. Try to find out what her worries or concerns are. It is possible that she is not taking her asthma treatment or that she needs a different treatment.

We suggest your daughter has a check-up with the asthma nurse or doctor to review how well controlled her asthma is. She may prefer to talk to the asthma nurse or doctor without you being present during the consultation.

### Why does cold weather make me cough? Is there anything I can do to help this?

Changes in weather and temperature are known to trigger asthma symptoms. For some people, breathing in cold air results in airway spasm or tightness. Others find that cold weather can cause coughing as well. Damp or wet weather or even hot weather can also make the airways react and become tight.

Why don't you make an appointment to see your asthma nurse or doctor? You need to make sure that you are taking the right asthma medicines, in the right dose to control your asthma symptoms and in the right inhaler device.

Do use your blue inhaler (reliever) before you go out in the cold weather – you will find it helpful. You can also wrap up well with a scarf around your neck, covering your nose and mouth. This helps to warm the air before you breathe it in. The 'old wives tale' of wrapping up well in cold weather is really quite sensible!

### Why does the cold weather make me wheeze?

Breathing in cold air often makes people wheeze and cough, and can sometimes trigger dramatic asthma symptoms. This is more likely to happen if the air is dry as well as cold. Cold air is one of the inhaled irritants that can make your airways 'twitchy'. This tendency to twitchiness is called bronchial hyperreactivity (BHR). (See also the previous answer on coughing and cold weather.)

You can minimize your wheezing in cold weather by taking regular preventer asthma medicines and, if necessary, using extra reliever treatment before you go out into the cold air. This will help you to keep your asthma under good control. (See *Medicines* in Chapter 4.)

## What is passive smoking and why is it bad for you?

*Passive smoking* is breathing in air polluted by cigarette smoke from other people. Passive smoking is bad for you because it can irritate your airways even if you do not have asthma. If you have asthma, passive smoking is likely to make your asthma worse and cause increased asthma symptoms. Pubs, clubs and restaurants are more aware of the risks of passive smoking – smoking bans in these places are increasing.

## When I am in a smoky atmosphere I cough. Why?

A smoky atmosphere means that you breathe in things that irritate your airways. Cigarette smoke contains many chemicals and small particles that irritate the airways when you breathe them in. This is what we know as passive smoking.

It is definitely best to avoid smoky atmospheres as much as possible, especially if you have asthma, but it is not always possible, and we realize it is much easier said than done. It is recognized by health experts that passive smoking is potentially harmful and there are increasing laws to ban smoking in public places.

## When I tried to buy some aspirin, the chemist asked me if I had asthma. Why?

We know that certain medicines can make asthma worse. The most important group of these medicines is called the non-steroidal anti-inflammatory drugs (or *NSAIDs*); aspirin is one of these. Similar medicines include: ibuprofen, Nurofen, Junifen, indomethacin, Voltarol and diclofenac. Not everybody is aspirin sensitive but the pharmacist is quite right in being cautious. People with *nasal polyps* (swellings in the nose) are more likely to react to these medicines and therefore they should avoid taking them. Aspirin and the other NSAIDs can cause serious, sometimes life-threatening, asthma attacks in about 1 in 10 adults with asthma.

As you are probably aware, aspirin and many of the other NSAIDs are available without prescription and can be purchased in the supermarket or local pharmacy. These medicines are taken by lots of people in the UK for a range of complaints. These include: headache, period pains, joint pain and other aches and pains. Aspirin is also taken every day (in a low dose) by those at risk of stroke or heart attack. Aspirin should not be given to any child under the age of 16 because of potentially very serious reactions, such as *Reye's syndrome*. Allergic reactions to NSAIDs are rare in children.

### Are there any other medicines that affect asthma?

Although aspirin and NSAIDs are the most commonly used medicines to interfere with asthma, there are other important medicines such as *beta-blockers* that can make asthma worse or even trigger asthma symptoms. Beta-blocker medicines are used to treat high blood pressure and heart problems but they are also available as eye drops for the treatment of glaucoma. There are alternatives to these medicines and eye drops. Do talk to your asthma nurse or doctor or to your local pharmacist if you need advice.

### I have asthma. If I can't take aspirin, is it OK to take paracetamol?

Yes it is, but there have been some reports that asthma is made worse if you take paracetamol. The Department of Health has looked carefully at the use of paracetamol by people with asthma. From the evidence they have, the advice is that paracetamol is safe to take. However, if you feel that your asthma is made worse by paracetamol you should not take it. Do talk to your local pharmacist or your asthma nurse or doctor about alternative pain relief.

### How can I find out what makes my asthma worse if the cause is not obvious?

It is not always easy to find out what triggers asthma. One reason for this is that an allergic reaction to an asthma trigger may not occur until a number of hours after the exposure. This is known as a *late reaction* (rather than an immediate reaction), and makes it more difficult to spot the connection between contact with a trigger and symptoms.

Sometimes identifying what triggers your asthma is relatively easy. For example, if you have had a previous late reaction after being in contact with dogs, it can be fairly obvious what the trigger is, especially if you react some hours after you come into contact with a dog again. However, having multiple allergies (and therefore triggers) is quite common, particularly if you are atopic. Sometimes you have to be a bit of a detective to identify the asthma triggers. Skin tests may be helpful in identifying if you have an allergic response to certain triggers, but these tests only confirm an atopic tendency and not asthma itself. (See the questions about extrinsic and intrinsic asthma, and about allergy, in Chapter 3.)

If you develop asthma in adult life, viral infections are the most likely trigger. Allergic triggers are less likely, unless you have developed occupational asthma. (See the question **What is occupational asthma?** in Chapter 6.)

### Do different triggers affect different people?

Yes, but most people with asthma respond to a small number of common trigger factors. Everyone's airways (including people who do not suffer from asthma) will react to certain inhaled irritants. For example, people may cough when they go into a smoky room or when a crumb goes down the wrong way.

Allergic asthma, which is also known as atopic asthma, means that your airways have 'overreacted' to asthma allergens. These allergens are things that you have breathed in and are usually well-known substances. These substances include house dust mite, grass pollens and animal fur or hair, but there are many others. Particular allergens may trigger off a dramatic narrowing of the airways in someone with allergic asthma, causing wheezing, chest tightness and coughing.

Other people with asthma respond to different triggers such as virus infections, fumes, air pollution, exercise, cold air and laughter. These triggers are not allergens.

**My husband keeps me awake with his snoring. Is there likely to be any connection with his asthma?**

There may well be a connection between his snoring and asthma. A number of people do find that night-time asthma symptoms such as coughing result in snoring. The nose and the back of the throat can become quite swollen especially if there are symptoms such as a blocked nose, coughing or wheezing.

Sometimes respiratory symptoms cause a condition called 'obstructive sleep apnoea'. This means that the air passages become completely blocked especially when you are asleep, and you stop breathing for a short while before restarting with a noisy snore. This type of breathing can be very noisy and very disruptive to a normal sleep pattern. This may be the case with your husband and if so he would benefit from a consultation with his GP to discuss possible referral to a specialist.

**Why should the smell from a wood shop or a sawmill start off my attacks?**

Wood dust is an asthma trigger for some people, and you may be one of them. It is usually the fine wood dust found in sawmills or in industrial wood cutting, rather than the coarse sawdust associated with general building work. Medium density fibreboard, or MDF as we usually call it, is often used for making shelves, kitchen units and other furniture. When MDF is sawn or sanded the wood dust is very fine. This enables the wood dust to be breathed in easily and it reaches the smaller airways because of the size of the dust particles.

It is likely that the fine wood dust, and not the smell, starts off your attack. If you are close enough to smell the wood, you are close enough to inhale the dust. Have a look at the questions dealing with occupational asthma. (See the question **What is occupational asthma?** in Chapter 6.)

## Can 'living flame' gas fires make my asthma worse?

We are not aware of any published information specifically on 'living flame' gas fires. It seems likely that a 'living flame' gas fire is no different from any other gas fire in terms of pollution or fumes. Any gas fire is more likely to cause a problem if it is old or has not been properly serviced. Do make sure you have the fire checked regularly to make sure that it is safe and not producing any dangerous fumes. When the fire is lit the air temperature and humidity in the room will change. These changes in air temperature and humidity are quite potent triggers of asthma symptoms.

If your asthma is made worse when the fire is on, do make an appointment to see your asthma nurse or doctor. Poor asthma control will mean that your airways react very easily to irritants such as the gas fire.

Research has linked the use of 'biomass' fuels and increased asthma symptoms. These fuels are used for cooking indoors in many countries and there are current developments in the United Kingdom where biomass fuel crops are being grown. If you have asthma, it may not be advisable to use these fuels (see *Appendix*).

## I always get attacks in winter. Why is this?

There are several possible reasons but here are the three most likely:

- Your attacks probably result from a cold which goes on to your chest. An upper respiratory tract infection (common cold) is responsible, and is the most common asthma trigger. In the winter months there are more of these viral infections around than at any other time of year.

- Cold air is an important trigger factor and, of course, this will affect your chest more in the winter than at other times of the year.

- Finally, house dust mite numbers are at their highest in the early part of the winter, when the heating is switched on. If you are allergic to house dust mite, this may be the cause.

**I am 42 years old, and have a part-time job. When I am overtired, I tend to get an asthma attack. Why is this?**

Being overtired in itself does not cause you to have an asthma attack, but there are reasons why this might seem to be the case. Asthma can be triggered by many different things. It is possible that, when you are overtired or stressed, this plays an important role. You may feel very tired after you have exercised or you feel 'run down' while suffering from a cold or a virus infection. Exercise and virus infections are well-known asthma triggers.

When your asthma is poorly controlled, you may not be sleeping very well. People sometimes don't realize that their asthma is getting worse because it happens gradually over a period of time. They may adjust and cope with their symptoms until things become quite bad. If you are one of these people, it is more likely that worsening asthma is causing your tiredness, rather than the other way round.

**My asthma is caused by allergies. Why do I have attacks when I get excited or upset?**

Just because your asthma is mainly triggered by allergies, it does not mean that other trigger factors cannot cause symptoms, or even asthma attacks. Colds or other virus infections often make asthma worse, but around 40% of people with asthma report that emotional stress or overexcitement can make their asthma worse. If your asthma is not under control, these things are more likely to affect you. On the other hand, if your asthma is under control, you are less likely to get symptoms that are related to stress.

**Why do some things such as cat hairs trigger off my asthma symptoms, but similar things such as dog hairs do not?**

We do not know the complete answer here. There is so much variation between individuals that it becomes impossible to cover all the factors involved.

Not everyone is allergic to the same substances and just what triggers off your asthma will depend on your particular allergy.

Domestic pets often live close to us and their hair or feathers can trigger asthma symptoms.

Cats are the most common trigger of animal allergy, particularly in children. Many people are allergic only to kittens, or to certain breeds, particularly Siamese and Burmese. Dogs, horses, hamsters and guineapigs can also cause allergic asthma.

Although hair and shed skin are often responsible for the allergy, surprisingly it has been shown that the allergen is in a cat's saliva. When the animal washes itself, the allergen sticks to hairs allowing easier contact with the person with asthma.

**My asthma is worse just before my period. Is there any connection?**

Yes, there may be. Hormonal changes are known to have an effect on asthma in some people. Asthma symptoms are often worse immediately before a period. If you think your periods are having an influence on your asthma control, record your peak flow readings twice daily (morning and evening) for 2–3 months. You will then be able to see the pattern of your blowing tests and establish if your tests are worse just before a period and whether these really do influence your asthma control. (See the sections covering peak expiratory flow in Chapters 3 and 5.) If you think your asthma is not under control, do go and talk to your asthma nurse or doctor and take any peak flow readings with you – it may help to identify what is making your asthma worse. If your asthma is under control, you are less likely to notice any hormonal influences. (See the section on *Sex, periods, pregnancy and the menopause* in Chapter 6.)

**My asthma was awful during my last pregnancy. Why?**

During pregnancy there are many changes in hormone levels and unfortunately some people with asthma do find that their asthma gets worse. It is really important that you continue your asthma treatment even though you are pregnant. If your asthma is not under control, it is more likely to be harmful to your baby than taking your asthma medicines. Asthma medicines are safe and should be taken as usual, even taking a course of *steroid* tablets if it is needed. It is difficult to predict what your asthma will be like during any subsequent pregnancies, although some people do report similar patterns. (See the section on ***Sex, periods, pregnancy and the menopause*** in Chapter 6.)

## All in the mind?

### Is my asthma really psychological?

If you mean 'Is my asthma all in my mind?', the answer is definitely no. However, certain psychological factors such as stress can trigger asthma attacks. This happens in people who already have asthma in the first place.

It is important to be aware that asthma can have a strong psychological effect on sufferers and their families. Most people with asthma need to take regular medication and, if they forget, they may become unwell. Even if they do take regular treatment, they may still get an occasional severe attack. These attacks may start suddenly without warning and this can be very stressful to the whole family. Some families have experience of really bad asthma attacks – holidays spoilt and lack of sleep. These things have a major effect on their lives. Regular monitoring (see Chapters 5 and 6) and effective treatment (see Chapter 4) will reduce these problems and the amount of stress that they might cause.

### Are nervous people more prone to asthma?

No. However, there are some asthma symptoms that some people associate with nervous problems. Breathlessness is sometimes seen as a sign of nervousness but this sometimes happens in people who do not have asthma.

Life with asthma can be very unpredictable. Asthma can vary from day to day – one day all will be well, and on another an acute asthma attack may occur. This is enough to make anyone nervous or anxious. Research has shown that severe asthma in children is associated with depression in mothers. What comes first? Does the depressed mother make her child more likely to develop asthma, or does the fact that her child has severe asthma cause depression in the mother? We don't know for sure.

### My mum died when I was 10 years old. Shortly afterwards I developed asthma. Could some other serious upset cause it to go away?

It may have seemed as if your mum's death was the cause of your asthma but there may have been others. Asthma is an unpredictable condition. There are many reasons why it begins, and just as many for its disappearance. Probably a combination of circumstances is needed for the asthma to appear at this time, but the other factors may be less obvious. It is less likely that further trauma will cause it to go away.

### I have asthma and when my children were born I had postnatal depression. I have heard that asthma is a nervous condition so is there a link?

We do not believe that asthma is a nervous condition. However, it is accepted that depression can make some people's asthma worse. It is important to remember that depression on its own will not cause asthma in someone who has never had it before. Both conditions are very common. Asthma occurs in approximately 5% of the adult population, and postnatal depression affects around 10% of women in the year after childbirth. So it is not surprising that the two conditions occur together in some cases. However, there is no important link between asthma and postnatal depression. Mothers with and without asthma have an equal chance of developing it.

### Is stress in my marriage responsible for the poor control of my asthma?

There is no doubt that, in some people, stress and other psychological factors can make asthma worse and can lead to constant symptoms. For most people, emotional stresses have little or no effect on asthma. There are often several trigger factors that occur at the same time, and emotional upset may be just one of them. The stress in your marriage may be contributing to your poor asthma control, but we doubt whether it is the only cause. Rather than just putting up with your asthma symptoms, do go and see your asthma nurse or doctor to see if your symptom control can be improved so that there will be one less problem for you to deal with.

**I suffer from claustrophobia. Is this usual for people with asthma?**

Not really. Claustrophobia is the fear of closed or confined spaces. It is very unpleasant and quite common, though not as common as asthma, and some people do suffer from both conditions. Many people feel panicky during an asthma attack and often feel the need to find open space and fresh air.

Asthma is so common that many people with other conditions as well will question whether these are linked to their asthma. Usually there will not be a link (but see the next section).

# *Related conditions*

**Are there any ailments or illnesses associated with asthma?**

Yes – there are two conditions that are closely associated with asthma. These are:

- hay fever (allergic rhinitis)

- eczema.

People with two or three of these conditions (asthma, hay fever or eczema) are known as atopic individuals.

There are other conditions that are less common, but also related to asthma, including:

- polyps (small fleshy, non-cancerous growths) in the nose

- allergic skin conditions such as urticaria – this consists of raised blotchy patches on the skin looking very much like nettle rash.

People with true, diagnosed food allergy and asthma are more at risk of having a severe attack of asthma. If you have both of these conditions, it is really wise to make sure you go for regular check-ups with your asthma nurse or doctor.

Other important chronic conditions, such as high blood pressure and diabetes are not directly related to asthma. They often occur in those with asthma because they are also common.

### How do I know it's asthma and not allergy?

Asthma and allergy are very closely related. Allergy occurs when the body reacts against an external substance. The allergic response can start as an asthma attack or an episode of uncontrolled asthma but asthma is not the only response. An allergic response can trigger symptoms such as a runny nose, a skin rash or swollen eyelids. There are lots of things that can cause an allergic response, such as pollen, dust or even medicines such as penicillin.

### What should I tell my asthma nurse or doctor about my asthma symptoms?

Talking to your asthma nurse or doctor about your asthma symptoms will help you check if your asthma is under control. Do explain how your asthma affects your life especially if it is preventing you from doing things. Monitoring asthma symptoms should be part of an action or management plan. Do discuss this with your asthma nurse or doctor so that you know exactly what to look for. Coughing, wheezing, chest tightness or shortness of breath are all signs that your asthma is not under control.

**Personal action plan – things you might wish to discuss with your doctor or asthma nurse**

- If you are having more respiratory symptoms than usual, your asthma is not under good control. Night-time symptoms are particularly important pointers to this. Do make an appointment for an asthma check-up.

- Many asthma triggers are difficult to avoid. Talk to your doctor or asthma nurse about your asthma triggers to see if anything can be done to help you reduce your exposure to them.

- Smoking can make asthma worse and cause long-term health problems. If you smoke and want help to stop smoking, do go and talk to your doctor, asthma nurse or pharmacist for advice and support. There are various smoking cessation aids such as nicotine gum and patches that can help you.

- If you find your asthma symptoms are better when you are away from work or on holiday, it is possible you have occupational or work-aggravated asthma. Discuss this with your health professional.

- When you next see your doctor or asthma nurse, you might want to find out if you are taking the right asthma medicines. Recording peak flow readings twice a day for 2 weeks and charting them will help to assess your asthma control. Take these peak flow readings with you when you go to the surgery.

# 3
# How is asthma diagnosed?

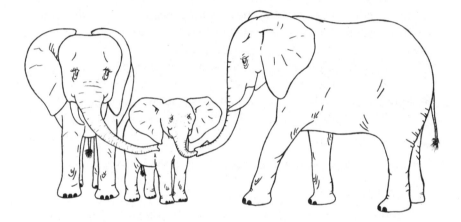

In this chapter you will learn about:

- how asthma is diagnosed

- the symptoms of asthma

- how it affects people

- how to look after yourself if you have asthma

- how to know when asthma is getting worse

- how to prevent asthma attacks

- other respiratory (breathing) conditions that may be confused with asthma.

When people go to see a health professional with breathing problems, it suggests that there is a respiratory (lung) cause. Breathing problems are called respiratory symptoms and are mainly:

- coughing

- wheezing

- shortness of breath.

These symptoms are often due to infections caused by colds. Colds are the result of virus infections and in most people they get better without any treatment in 1–2 weeks.

The main question doctors and asthma nurses need to answer when someone consults is whether respiratory symptoms are caused by an infection such as a cold, or due to something that is non-infectious such as asthma. If you have an infection you may:

- feel ill quite quickly

- have a temperature or fever

- have a runny nose

- sometimes cough up phlegm, which is thick and sticky and a greenish colour.

Asthma is very variable and it affects people in different ways. For some, asthma symptoms happen only if they have a cold, and the symptoms clear up once the cold has gone. This is known as 'episodic asthma'. Symptoms such as coughing or wheezing are more troublesome when others are exposed to things that cause their asthma to flare up. The many things that cause this are known as asthma triggers. For example, asthma is frequently triggered by a lot of pollen in the air such as in the 'hay fever' season. In other cases, asthma gets worse if there is exposure to other triggers such as dust, smoky atmospheres or strong smells.

Making the diagnosis of asthma can be difficult, but the main clue is that the symptoms come and go, often very frequently. Chest infections do not recur so often in the same person; anyone needing to see a doctor or asthma nurse more than two or three times a year for repeated respiratory symptoms is likely to have asthma, until proved otherwise.

Some people have an inherited chance of developing asthma. The clue to this is whether there is a family medical history of asthma. A family history of asthma, or other allergic conditions such as hay fever (allergic rhinitis), eczema, allergy to food or medicines (such as penicillin or other antibiotics), means that there is a greater risk of developing any of these conditions.

# When should asthma be suspected?

## Clues to diagnosis

As stated previously, when people consult their doctor frequently with symptoms of cough, wheeze and shortness of breath, asthma should be considered as a diagnosis. 'Cold symptoms' that go on for weeks and weeks could in fact be due to asthma.

These symptoms are often worse at night and more persistent in people with asthma. They often carry on coughing or wheezing for more than 6 weeks when they have a virus infection, whereas for those without asthma a virus infection, even if it causes coughing and wheezing, will clear up much more quickly. Coughing or wheezing that is made worse by laughing or exercise also suggests underlying asthma.

People with occupational asthma, or asthma that is caused by exposure to substances at work, are often better when away from their work environment. The question asked by health professionals to diagnose this condition is: '**Are your symptoms of coughing or wheezing better when you are away from work or on holiday?**' If this is the case, then you should discuss the problem with your occupational health adviser at work, or your general practitioner or asthma nurse.

**How can I find out what triggers my asthma if the cause is not obvious?**

We have listed the common trigger factors for asthma symptoms in Chapter 2 of this book. However, it is not always easy for you to find out what is the most important trigger for your asthma. One reason for this is that the reaction to a trigger may come after many hours (known as a 'late reaction'), rather than immediately. This makes it more difficult to make the connection between coming into contact with a trigger, and your asthma.

A daily symptom diary chart is an ideal way for you to find out about your particular triggers. These charts are available from your doctor or asthma nurse and may be helpful. It may be best to draw a chart specially marked with possible triggers for your own particular situation. This can be done by taking a page of graph paper and marking it as shown in Figure 3.1.

We have suggested some of the possible trigger factors. You may wish to add others. For example:

- If you go horse riding, add this to your chart.

- Write down any symptoms that start in the few days after going horse riding.

- Mark your chart daily, using a 'Y' for yes when you have come up against the possible trigger.

- Compare this chart with your asthma symptoms; it may be possible to identify a pattern indicating which triggers are responsible.

In addition to a peak flow chart, a symptom chart may provide extra information on possible triggers of your asthma. You will find more information about taking peak flow readings and keeping charts in Chapter 5 in the section *Peak expiratory flow monitoring*.

Having given you all this information, we have to admit that for some people, particularly those whose asthma starts in adult life, it may prove impossible to find a clearly identifiable trigger. Regardless of a trigger you are left needing to control your asthma as effectively as possible with treatment.

| Date | | | | | | | |
|---|---|---|---|---|---|---|---|
| Symptoms | | | | | | | |
| Cough | | | | | | | |
| Wheeze | | | | | | | |
| Shortness of breath | | | | | | | |
| Peak flow | | | | | | | |
| 650 | | | | | | | |
| 600 | | | | | | | |
| 550 | | | | | | | |
| 500 | | | | | | | |
| 450 | | | | | | | |
| 400 | | | | | | | |
| 350 | | | | | | | |
| 300 | | | | | | | |
| 250 | | | | | | | |
| 200 | | | | | | | |
| 150 | | | | | | | |
| 100 | | | | | | | |
| 50 | | | | | | | |
| Worked today | | | | | | | |
| Exercised today | | | | | | | |
| Decorated house | | | | | | | |
| Cleaned house | | | | | | | |
| Worked with dust | | | | | | | |
| Worked in garden | | | | | | | |
| Caught cold | | | | | | | |
| Tried a different food | | | | | | | |

**Figure 3.1** Daily symptom diary chart.

# *Diagnosis of asthma – tests and investigations*

Once asthma is suspected by a doctor or asthma nurse, the diagnosis needs to be confirmed. This is so that:

- treatment can be prescribed

- an action plan for managing asthma can be agreed between you and the doctor or asthma nurse.

Knowing how to prevent an asthma attack can also be discussed once the diagnosis has been made.

There are three ways of confirming the diagnosis of asthma:

- from the clues in the person's medical history – their symptoms and when they occur

- by prescribing an anti-asthma medicine and seeing if the symptoms improve

- by doing tests that identify whether the airways are becoming narrow (obstructed) during periods of respiratory symptoms.

The diagnosis of asthma is more likely if the person also suffers from allergy, eczema or hay fever, or if there are people in the family who also have these conditions.

## How do doctors diagnose asthma?

There is more than one way of diagnosing asthma. The medical history on its own is often enough for the diagnosis to be made. There are many factors in the past medical history to suggest asthma as the cause of someone's problem.

Asthma is a chronic (long-lasting) condition, in which people may be free from symptoms for periods of time and very ill at others. They will usually have a pattern of symptoms that come and go.

In asthma the symptoms often get worse with exercise, laughter, colds, or when in a smoky or dusty room. Anyone who has frequent coughs, or who gets wheezy frequently, should be suspected of having asthma until proved otherwise.

The diagnosis can be confirmed by the health professional by two methods. One way is to see if anti-asthma medication clears the symptoms. Sometimes this may need to be taken for weeks before it starts to work. In young children this is the most suitable way of making the diagnosis, together with a detailed medical history. A more convincing way in older children and adults is by the use of peak flow meter readings or more detailed blowing tests called *spirometry*.

# Blowing tests: peak expiratory flow and spirometry

Asthma is a condition that causes narrowing of the airways, due to:

- spasm of the muscle surrounding the airways

- swelling of the airway walls

- increased mucus inside the airways.

Tests used to diagnose asthma and to see if the airways are narrowed are:

- the *peak expiratory flow* test (also known as the peak flow or PEF)

- spirometry.

Peak flow meters are relatively inexpensive and are available on prescription; they are very useful for diagnosing and checking on asthma. Use of spirometers requires quite a lot of training and they are usually used by doctors and asthma nurses to diagnose lung diseases other than asthma. Both of these tests are used to measure how tight the airways are and to see if the tightness improves after treatment. The tighter (or narrower) the airways are, the lower the peak flow or spirometry readings.

These tests are also used to obtain blowing measurements or readings, during episodes when people have symptoms, and at times when there are none. In someone without asthma, the readings stay almost the same. Asthma is confirmed if the PEF readings change (vary) by more than 20% from morning to evening or day to day.

There are three main patterns of peak flow charts suggestive of asthma: these are shown in Figures 3.2, 3.3, 3.4 and 3.5. Figure 3.6 shows how readings can be recorded without using graphs.

The peak expiratory flow is a measurement of how air flows through the airways in the lungs. If the airways are narrowed, as in episodes of asthma, then the readings are lower. In asthma, peak

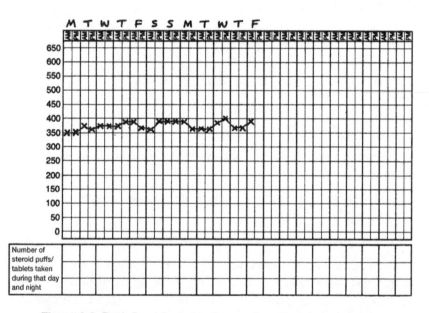

**Figure 3.2** Peak flow chart showing readings that do not change from day to day. This type of chart is seen either in people who have well-controlled asthma at this time or those who do not have asthma.

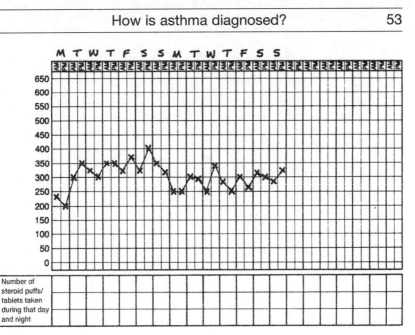

**Figure 3.3** Peak flow chart showing changing readings (variation) from day to day. In someone with symptoms of asthma, a chart like this would help to confirm the diagnosis of asthma. In someone with asthma, this chart indicates poor control and more treatment is needed.

flow readings can vary between good times and bad times by more than 20%. If this is demonstrated, then the diagnosis of asthma is confirmed. The blowing test can take place during the consultation with the doctor or asthma nurse but you may be asked to keep a 'peak flow diary' at home.

The important changes that will help doctors and asthma nurses to diagnose asthma from the peak flow diary results are:

- a variation between readings of more than 20%

- an increased difference between the morning and evening readings

- an early *morning dip* in the readings.

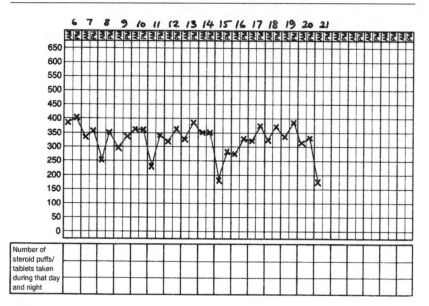

**Figure 3.4** Peak flow chart showing early morning dipping in the readings. In someone with symptoms of asthma, a chart like this would help to confirm the diagnosis of asthma. In someone with asthma, this chart indicates poor control and more treatment is needed.

## How are the changes (variation) in peak flow readings worked out?

The changes in peak flow readings can be worked out by the following simple mathematical equation:

$$\frac{\text{Highest PEF reading} - \text{lowest PEF reading}}{\text{Highest PEF reading}} \times 100 = \text{\% change in PEF}$$

In the peak flow chart in Figure 3.7:

- the highest PEF reading is 400; the lowest PEF reading is 300.

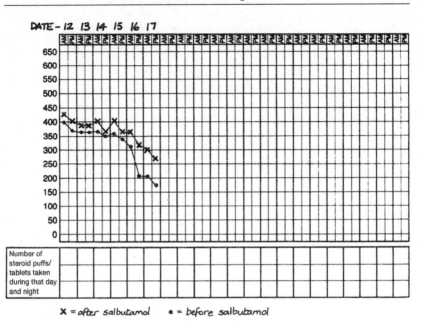

x = after salbutamol    • = before salbutamol

**Figure 3.5** Peak flow chart showing readings that are dropping from day to day. This person has poorly controlled, deteriorating asthma. Urgent help is needed.

Using the above calculation:

$$\frac{\text{Highest PEF reading (400)} - \text{lowest PEF reading (300)}}{\text{Highest PEF reading (400)}} \times 100 = 25\% \text{ change in PEF}$$

Put even more simply:

$$\frac{400 - 300}{400} \times 100 = \frac{100}{400} = 25\% \text{ change in PEF}$$

In this example, the variation between the highest and lowest readings is 25%, confirming the diagnosis of asthma.

| Day | Morning readings (best of 3) | Evening readings (best of 3) |
|---|---|---|
| Monday 25th | 230 | 200 |
| Tuesday 26th | 300 | 350 |
| Wednesday 27th | 300 | 330 |
| Thursday 28th | 350 | 350 |
| Friday 29th | 330 | 370 |
| Saturday 30th | 320 | 400 |
| Sunday 31st | 350 | 320 |
| Monday 1st | 250 | 250 |
| Tuesday 2nd | 300 | 290 |
| Wednesday 3rd | 250 | 340 |
| Thursday 4th | 280 | 250 |

**Figure 3.6** Some people are not familiar with graphs. This child's family have recorded her peak flow readings using numbers. These change from day to day, from 200 to 350 litres/minute. She probably has asthma.

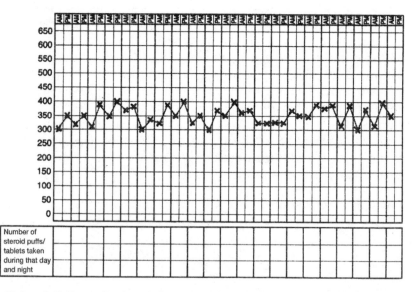

**Figure 3.7** Example of peak flow chart showing change of over 20% in the readings. This chart helps to confirm the diagnosis of asthma.

## How do peak flow readings help diagnose asthma?

The response to anti-asthma treatment can be assessed by asking people if they are better and by recording and charting peak flow readings.

- If anti-asthma medication makes you better, you may have asthma – sometimes this medicine needs to be continued for quite a few weeks, or even months, before it starts to work.

- If the peak expiratory flow improves with treatment, this confirms the diagnosis of asthma.

On a peak flow chart, three things to watch for to see if there are any improvements are:

- an increase in the readings (this should be at least 20% for the diagnosis to be confirmed)

- a decreased gap between the morning and evening readings

- a great reduction in early morning dips in the readings.

Figure 3.8 shows two of these things. This man saw his doctor on the 6th of the month. The doctor confirmed the diagnosis of asthma from the medical history and started treatment with an inhaled steroid at two puffs twice a day. The man was asked to keep a record of his morning and evening peak flow readings. The graph shows the improvement in readings, which gradually increase from 300 to around 500. The gap between the morning and evening readings gets less during the following weeks and the readings level off after about 4 weeks.

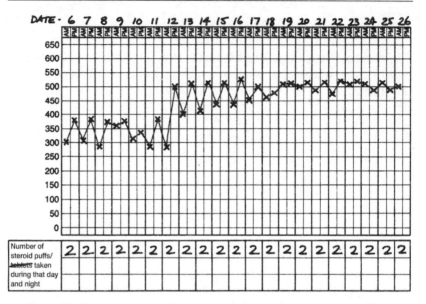

Figure 3.8 Peak flow chart showing a gradual improvement in readings after starting inhaler treatment for asthma.

# Is it really asthma, and is there more than one type?

### Have I really got asthma?

A lot of people ask this question, especially if they have only mild or occasional symptoms. Many believe that to have asthma you need to be quite poorly and quite limited when doing everyday things. This is not always true and, in fact, most people with asthma have mild asthma.

There are certain pointers that will establish whether or not you really do have asthma. The story you tell the doctor about the nature and frequency of your symptoms and what brings them on should alert him or her to the diagnosis. You may well be asked to blow into a peak flow meter for a week or so, and to record your measurements twice a day. Your doctor or asthma nurse will be looking to see how much your readings vary between the morning and the evening, and from day to day. If they vary by 20% or more asthma is by far the most likely cause.

Another way of confirming that you really do have asthma is for your doctor or asthma nurse to measure your peak flow before and after exercise or treatment (exercise testing or reversibility testing). We need to be careful with interpreting these tests because, although a positive result confirms asthma, if they are not conclusive they do not necessarily rule it out.

## Do different people have different types of asthma, or is it all the same?

This question is in two parts, and really there are two ways of answering it. In one sense, all people with asthma have the same condition. They have that combination of twitchy airways and overproduction of mucus from swollen airway linings, which leads to the symptoms of asthma. However, there is an enormous range of asthma among different people. The speed with which the condition develops, the triggers that continue to provoke it, and the responses to different treatments all vary widely between individuals.

Asthma can be categorized in different ways:

- allergic or non-allergic according to what usually triggers episodes

- mild, moderate or severe, according to the seriousness of the episodes

- easy, difficult or brittle, according to the way it responds to treatments.

One form of asthma, which is sometimes regarded as a different condition, is 'occupational asthma', because it is more clearly defined in terms of its cause. This is asthma that starts as a result of something in the workplace and that people do not come up against anywhere else. A good example of occupational asthma is that caused by fumes from soldering work in the electronics industry. This is the only curable form of asthma, provided it is diagnosed early and the person is no longer exposed to the causative agents (allergens). This does not mean that the person should lose their job. Rather it means that the employer should try to provide a clean environment for the worker, where (s)he is not exposed to the offending agent.

**My doctor has diagnosed viral-associated wheeze in my 3-year-old son? What does he mean by that – I thought he had asthma?**

You have obviously mentioned to your doctor that your son's wheezing is triggered by colds. It is quite normal for preschool children to have about six or seven colds every year, but in some children the cold virus sets off chest symptoms, one of which is wheezing. Viral-associated wheeze (also referred to as VAW by some doctors) is wheezing, which is triggered only by viral infections. It is likely that viral wheezing is a type of mild asthma.

What you tell your doctor about your son's wheezing will help to 'paint the picture' as to what is happening and help your doctor to decide on the right treatment. Although your doctor has not confirmed the diagnosis of asthma in your son, asthma reliever inhaler medicines are helpful in treating wheezing. If the viral wheezing is very bad and your son's breathing is difficult, we sometimes need to give a short course of steroid tablets for a few days to get over the crisis period. In addition your son will need an inhaler medicine (the blue reliever inhaler) to 'open up' and relax the airways, so the air can get in and out more easily when he breathes.

Unfortunately, asthma can be difficult to diagnose in this age group because blowing tests cannot be carried out – the technique of blowing is just not possible. If your son continues to wheeze with colds, simple blowing tests with a peak flow meter will help to confirm the diagnosis of asthma when he is about 6 years of age.

Viral wheezing often improves with age and in some children goes away altogether. If your child has eczema and a family history of asthma, asthma is easier to diagnose. We also know that in young children, a smoky environment increases respiratory viral infections. If you smoke, stopping smoking will really benefit you, your son and others around you.

**I have heard people talking about extrinsic and intrinsic asthma. What do they mean?**

We used to categorize asthma into one of two groups, called extrinsic and intrinsic. The problem with doing this is that there is often an overlap between the two. Nowadays we use the terms allergic and non-allergic asthma.

The most obvious feature about *extrinsic asthma* is that it is triggered by external or 'outside' allergens such as pollen and house dust mite. It tends to start in childhood and often occurs along with eczema and hay fever. If skin tests for allergy are carried out, they are positive to one or more of the common allergens. Symptoms of extrinsic asthma tend to come and go and sometimes the affected person is completely free of them.

*Intrinsic asthma* tends to start later in life, and skin tests, if they are carried out, are negative. Unfortunately, the symptoms are usually persistent and there may be no easily identifiable triggers, except for common colds. People with this type of asthma are sometimes sensitive to aspirin, and some develop small non-malignant (non-cancerous) growths in the nose called nasal polyps.

Many doctors regard this division into two types as unhelpful, because there may be such an overlap between the groups, with asthma sufferers showing features of both.

## What other diseases can be incorrectly diagnosed instead of asthma?

### Are there any ailments or illnesses associated with asthma?

Yes – there are three common and very important conditions that are closely associated with asthma. These are:

- eczema
- hay fever (allergic rhinitis)
- a general allergy to various things (for example, cats, dogs, horses, house dust mite and some medicines).

Another very important condition which may be difficult to separate from asthma is *chronic obstructive pulmonary disease* (COPD). In COPD, lung function tests such as spirometry do not usually improve, as they do in people with asthma. The two conditions often occur together, particularly in the elderly.

There are other conditions that are less common, but also related to asthma, including *polyps* (small non-cancerous growths) in the nose and allergic skin conditions such as urticaria. Urticaria consists of raised blotchy patches on the skin looking very much like nettle rash.

## Is my asthma an allergy?

Asthma and allergy are not the same, but asthma can be triggered by an allergic reaction to substances such as grass pollen, house dust mite and pet hair. If you have an allergy, it means that you are sensitive to ordinary everyday substances to which most people do not react.

For example, most people sneeze if pepper gets into their nose, and everyone's eyes will water if they peel onions. People with allergies will react in similar ways (getting itchy eyes, a runny nose or wheezing) if they come into contact with something to which they are allergic. For those allergic to cats, handling, stroking, or even being in the same room as one, will produce these symptoms.

Generally speaking an allergy develops over a long time and an allergic reaction does not happen the first time you come into contact with a substance. Some people's asthma is certainly triggered by an allergy. If you are one of these people and if the allergen can be found, then it would be sensible to avoid or reduce the amount of contact with the offending substance wherever possible. However, this may be easier said than done!

## How do I know it's asthma and not allergy?

Allergy occurs when the body reacts against an external substance. This might be pollen, dust or medicines, e.g. penicillin. The allergic reaction may take the form of a runny nose, a skin rash, swelling of the eyelids or wheezing. The allergic reaction may start an asthma attack or an episode of uncontrolled asthma. Allergy is one of the triggers of asthma and therefore may occur at the same time. The best way to tell if it is asthma is to use a peak flow chart, using the best of three readings in the morning and the evening (or more frequently if symptoms are bad). In asthma the peak flow goes up and down – it does not remain steady. By this we mean that the readings change from day to day, morning to evening or week to week. A variation of 20% or more shows that the asthma is out of control and is causing the symptoms (see the sections covering peak expiratory flow in Chapters 3 and 5).

## What is atopy?

Atopy is not a disease. Atopy means that the person reacts positively to skin prick tests to certain substances (like grass, cats or house dust mite). It is a part or feature of a person's genetic make-up that makes them liable to certain problems called allergic conditions. Being atopic does not mean that a person is allergic! When someone with atopy develops symptoms (for example, cough, sneeze or wheeze) when exposed to substances that cause them to react (like pollen), then they are diagnosed with allergy. One in three people in the UK suffers from allergy; the main conditions are asthma, eczema and hay fever. Therefore, to be atopic is to have inherited the tendency to these conditions. Not everyone who is atopic actually suffers from eczema, hay fever or asthma.

Genetic research suggests that the tendency to get asthma is inherited separately from the atopic tendency. However, if you have both, it is much more likely that you will develop asthma. That's why it is common for the three conditions of asthma, hay fever and eczema to exist together. Not all atopic people have asthma, and not all people with asthma are atopic (although around 75% are).

One way to tell whether a person is atopic or not is a test in which the skin is pricked through solutions of allergen. This is called *skin prick testing*. This test is not widely available in the National Health Service, mainly because GPs are not paid for doing this, and there are very few allergy clinics in the UK. In atopic people, skin prick tests will nearly always give a positive result (a raised wheal like a nettle sting). A very small number of people react badly to certain skin prick tests, and can experience an asthma attack. An alternative test where there is no likelihood of a bad reaction to the test is a special blood test called a RAST test. This gives the most accurate results and confirms specific allergies.

On its own, a positive test does not help in diagnosing the cause of a person's symptoms. The combination of a history linking exposure to the substance (called an allergen) and the development of symptoms, plus a positive test, provides the strongest evidence for the diagnosis.

### What is the connection between asthma and eczema? Is asthma a kind of internal eczema?

A large proportion of the population, perhaps up to 30%, are 'atopic', as described in the previous question. To be atopic is to have inherited a tendency to develop an allergy. The most common of these illnesses are eczema and hay fever. Asthma is an inherited condition very often associated with atopy. It is thought that asthma is more liable to appear if the person is also atopic. In other words, having one condition, atopy, makes the development of the other, asthma, more likely. Atopic eczema occurs particularly in children, and is very common. Inevitably, many children have both asthma and eczema. Your suggestion that asthma is a kind of internal eczema is a very good one. Eczema causes red, irritable, itchy inflamed skin. This is very much like the inflammation that occurs in the linings of the airways in asthma. So the two conditions are connected, and in many ways they are similar.

### How does asthma differ from other chest conditions and breathing difficulties?

Asthma is a condition in which symptoms are caused by narrowing of the airways which is **reversible**. This means that symptoms come and go, and for much of the time people with asthma are completely well. For example, athletes with asthma are able to perform at their peak when their asthma is well controlled. This is the main difference between asthma and other chest conditions.

**Chronic bronchitis** is another condition affecting the airways, but it is not reversible. Chronic obstructive pulmonary disease (COPD – a group of chest diseases that include emphysema and chronic bronchitis, and which is discussed in the next question) are both conditions that usually affect older adults, often those who have smoked for many years. These diseases are permanent and treatment is used to lessen the symptoms. They tend to be more severe than asthma, and less responsive to asthma treatments. These people often need oxygen and a form of therapy called pulmonary rehabilitation, which includes exercise, physiotherapy and occupational therapy.

**Cystic fibrosis** is an inherited condition where there is a problem with the proteins made by the body. This means that respiratory mucus is very sticky and it blocks up the air passages. Although cystic fibrosis is usually diagnosed soon after birth, symptoms are similar to asthma but the child is frequently unwell and often fails to thrive. All doctors are aware of this condition as it is the commonest inherited disease, and therefore they will refer the child urgently to a respiratory paediatrician who will arrange for special tests to be done, if they suspect cystic fibrosis. These tests include a 'sweat test' where the salt content of sweat is collected and measured. Parents of these children may report that they have noticed that their child 'tastes salty' when they kiss them. Fortunately neonatal screening for cystic fibrosis will become a routine test in the UK, and carried out as part of the heel prick blood test that is done in newborn babies.

**Air pollution** causes a lot of chest symptoms. Miners and other industrial workers who are exposed to lots of fumes and dust also suffer from problems with their chests; they often develop scar tissue in the lungs as well as emphysema. Passive smoking is responsible for a lot of chest illness, particularly COPD. Both air pollution and passive smoking worsen asthma.

**Heart disease** may cause difficulty in breathing. This usually results from the collection of fluid in the lungs when the heart is not pumping effectively. One form of this, acute heart failure, used to be known as 'cardiac asthma', but it is a completely different condition, and the term is hardly ever used these days.

**I have emphysema. What is it, and is it associated with asthma?**

Emphysema is congenital in some people (i.e. some people are born with it) as well as being caused by air pollution (such as cigarette smoke or from certain occupations). In emphysema, the walls of the air spaces in the lungs are damaged. These air spaces, called alveoli, are normally very elastic (stretchy). When air is breathed in, the lungs inflate, and they contract when air is breathed out. In emphysema, this elasticity is destroyed and the lungs become very large from overexpansion. The damaged areas of the lungs mean that oxygen and waste products are not able to move in and out of the bloodstream. As a result people with emphysema become short of oxygen and they become very breathless, tired and lethargic.

The relationship between emphysema and asthma is unclear. There is some evidence suggesting that, when asthma is severe and persistent (chronic), it causes scar tissue to form in the lungs. This scar tissue can damage the walls of the air spaces and passages and this may lead to emphysema. It is not known for sure why this scar tissue develops in asthma, but it is believed to be a result of the chronic inflammation that occurs. Most asthma experts now advise that treatments that reduce inflammation should be used regularly in order to try to avoid the development of scar tissue.

**In elderly people, is there a link between having asthma now, and having had TB in the past?**

There is no direct link between TB (tuberculosis) and asthma. In other words, if you have TB, you are no more likely than anyone else of your own age to get asthma. The only possible link is an indirect one.

TB occurs less often than in the past. It used to be very common and a major cause of early death before effective treatment was available. However, it is very worrying that once again more people seem to be developing TB. This disease is often associated with poverty and poor housing, which is perhaps a reason for the recent increase in numbers of people with TB in the UK. People who spend their first years of life in developing countries often have TB. The first contact with TB (called primary TB) usually occurs in childhood, and nearly always leaves a small scar in the lungs. This scar could provide the beginnings of more serious TB infection later in life. Quite a number of elderly people have the scars of healed primary TB in their lungs (this is rare in middle-aged and young people). This scar hardly ever gives rise to any symptoms or problems. However, one known trigger for 'awakening' old TB is treatment with steroids. These, of course, are often used in the treatment of severe episodes of asthma.

Anyone who has had TB in the past should tell their doctor about this, particularly if they also have asthma. It may be necessary to have regular chest X-rays if steroid tablets are required for asthma. It is rare and can only happen if the individual concerned has had TB in the past. TB is a very serious infection, but it can now be cured completely by tablets, as long as it is recognized.

---

**Personal action plan – things you might wish to discuss with your doctor or asthma nurse**

If you think you or your child may have asthma, there are a number of questions to ask your doctor or asthma nurse:

- Are my symptoms due to asthma?
- How can I confirm the diagnosis?
- Shall I keep a peak flow chart over a few weeks?
- Is it worth trying one of the asthma treatments to see if this helps my symptoms?

If your doctor or asthma nurse has diagnosed asthma in you or your child, then you might want to ask about the treatments available:

- What are the options for you?
- Which type of inhaler device is best for you?

People with newly diagnosed asthma will benefit from having a personalized action plan – ask your doctor or asthma nurse for one.

Do look at the internet for more information. Some useful sites are listed at the end of this book.

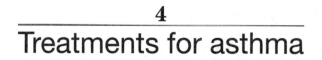

# 4
# Treatments for asthma

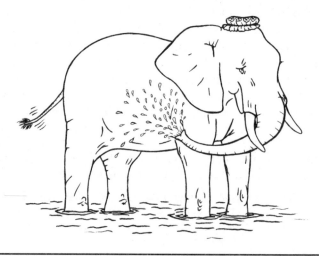

**In this chapter you will learn about:**

- how to reduce your (or your child's) exposure to asthma triggers

- the different sorts of complementary treatments that are sometimes tried by people with asthma

- why your asthma goes out of control and symptoms flare up

- the different medicines that are used to treat asthma

- the different inhaler devices that are available

- how to alter your asthma medicines to help control your asthma.

# Non-medicine treatments

## Allergen avoidance

**Is it possible to prevent allergic reactions? Does it help if you avoid exposure to allergens?**

People who have been sensitized to certain allergens may get allergic reactions when they come into contact with them. It makes sense for people to avoid the allergens that trigger their asthma, but of course this is not always possible.

How far do you go in trying to avoid allergens? Should you just try to reduce the particular allergen (or as many as possible) that cause symptoms? Research has shown that only reducing exposure to house dust mite in the home does not reduce asthma symptoms. However, most allergy specialists still advise people with asthma to try to reduce their exposure to as many allergens as possible, in order to reduce (rather than cure) their symptoms.

There is a wide range of allergy-reducing products that can be purchased. These products all make great claims that getting rid of allergens (mainly the house dust mite) from the home environment improves asthma. Some of them may be effective in reducing the number of house dust mites but do not necessarily improve asthma symptoms. Nearly all of the products are expensive, so we recommend that you get specialist advice before spending too much money in the hope of a miracle cure.

**My asthma is due to house dust. Would an air purifier or ionizer help?**

There are many preparations and devices claiming to reduce house dust mite levels, kill off the mites or purify the air.

**Air purifiers** may reduce the amount of dust in some areas of your home, but there is no proof that they help to improve asthma.

The air contains many tiny particles, which carry an electric charge, both positive and negative. **Ionizers** are machines that change positively charged particles in the air to negatively charged ones; this has the effect of removing them from the air. One research study found that an ionizer reduced the amount of house dust mites in the air in children's bedrooms, but there was no improvement in the children's symptoms. Another study showed that asthma symptoms were in fact made worse!

If you are thinking of buying one of these expensive devices, you may want to discuss it with someone. We suggest that you contact Asthma UK (address in *Appendix*) for more information.

Dust contains house dust mites, which can make your asthma considerably worse. You can reduce levels of dust in the home by:

- damp wiping areas that collect dust

- reducing the number of places or things that could collect dust, e.g. books, soft toys

- regular vacuum cleaning.

It is impossible to get rid of house dust mites completely. If you are allergic to house dust mites, it may be best to concentrate on reducing dust in the bedroom and living areas. Regular vacuuming of the mattress and sofas may help, but unfortunately special mattress covers alone, used as a single measure, have not been shown to be very effective. It may be worth trying a mixture of ways to reduce the house dust mite allergen, to see if it helps.

If dust makes your asthma worse, try to avoid places where major building or decorating work is being done.

**Is asthma aggravated by using a vacuum cleaner? There are some very expensive vacuum cleaners, which claim to help this problem. Are they effective?**

House dust and house dust mites are found in huge quantities in all carpets, cushions and bedding. However, it is the amount of dust and house dust mite allergen in the air (and in the bed mattress) that is important in determining symptoms.

Vacuuming disturbs the dust and leads to an increase in the amounts in the air, and can actually make the asthma worse – at least in the short term. Some preparations, including carpet shampoos, will kill off house dust mites; unfortunately, this is only a short-term solution as new dust mites will come back.

Some vacuum cleaners have special filters called HEPA filters (HEPA stands for high-efficiency particulate arrest). These types of filters within a vacuum cleaner help to trap very small particles of dust that would otherwise simply recirculate into the air during vacuuming. While vacuum cleaners with HEPA filters help to reduce dust, there is limited evidence as to whether they reduce allergens and therefore improve asthma symptoms. In addition these vacuum cleaners tend to be much more expensive (see Allergy UK in *Appendix*).

### My child has asthma. Should we have the cat put to sleep?

As you may guess from our response to this question, having the cat put to sleep is not a simple solution to the problem, even if you or your child has a true allergy to cats. Why don't you see if you can find an alternative home for your pet? We recommend that you discuss the question carefully with your doctor or asthma nurse. Removing a much-loved family pet sometimes causes so much upset that the asthma may become worse for a while.

Some people do find their asthma improves after a pet is removed from the home. However, the presence of a cat in the house may both cause asthma and protect someone from getting symptoms of asthma. The very presence of a cat in the house may even help to protect someone from reacting to cats. The theory of how this works is similar to the way we are immunized to certain diseases by having vaccinations (for example like tetanus, polio and diphtheria).

By being exposed to cat dander over a period of time the body gets used to (or immune to) the cat dander. This is why some people do not get asthma from cats even though they may be sensitized to them.

When this cat is removed from the house, the sensitized person still has the antibodies to cats in their bloodstream. When they are next exposed to cats, the antibodies react with the cat allergens to cause an asthma reaction.

Even after removal of a cat, asthma symptoms may persist for some time. Removal of a cat or any other pet from the home may help in the short term, but may cause more problems later. It is also the case that once one trigger has set off the asthma, other triggers may become equally important in keeping the symptoms there.

Washing or wiping the cat with a damp cloth once or twice a week may reduce the amount of cat allergen, but has very little impact on asthma symptoms – and washing or wiping the cat is easier said than done!

### Is it a good idea to try desensitizing treatments for specific allergies?

There are a few circumstances under which a specialist might advise *desensitization*. If your life is at risk from a severe allergy, such as to bee or wasp sting venom, desensitization is worthwhile. Others who may benefit from desensitization are those who have asthma in the summer months as a result of very severe hay fever, especially if is not improving with the usual treatment.

The treatment for these conditions is called immunotherapy and may last for several years. Desensitization involves injecting you with tiny amounts of the substance (e.g. grass pollen) to which you are allergic. This enables your body to build up a gradual resistance to the injected allergen.

This form of treatment is available only in specialist hospital centres but it can be very successful. It is very time consuming because frequent appointments are needed during the desensitization programme, and there are potentially some risks of a severe allergic reaction. For this reason, desensitization should only be carried out where there is emergency resuscitation equipment. Most people with asthma will not benefit from this sort of treatment and, instead, should try to reduce exposure to substances or animals that trigger their asthma attacks.

### Should I buy feather or synthetic pillows? Which is better from the point of view of reducing house dust mites?

It doesn't really matter what sort of pillow you have: house dust mites live in both types! What is important is the quality of the pillow cover; the smaller the weave of the cover the better. Feather pillows tend to have tightly woven covers and are therefore better for this reason. Buying new pillows every 5 years is an expense, but will probably help to reduce house dust mite exposure.

## Conventional mattresses obviously harbour the house dust mites. Are there any materials which are better for mattress construction?

Not for mattress construction, but there are some tightly woven mattress covering materials that do not allow the mites living in the mattress to escape. Polythene or plastic coverings can be used, but they tend to make the mattress hot and uncomfortable, and can be noisy whenever you roll over in bed. This can be annoying, particularly if sleep is already difficult because of asthma!

Some newer materials have pores that are too small for the mite to penetrate, but large enough for air to circulate to the mattress. Research has shown that these covers reduce the number of house dust mites; however, on their own they don't reduce asthma symptoms. Other measures are needed to reduce as many allergens as possible. Mattress covers are very expensive, but may be worth considering if you notice that your asthma is clearly related to dust allergy or if your nose becomes blocked. We know that allergy in the nose (allergic rhinitis) can also make asthma worse and nasal treatments may be required.

## Should I buy a mattress cover for my daughter's bed?

If your daughter's asthma is caused by dust allergy it may be worth trying a special mattress cover. Before you spend lots of money on covers to reduce house dust mite exposure, it is worth confirming that your daughter is actually allergic to house dust mite. Simple tests such as skin prick tests or blood tests can do this, and may be available in your general practice.

If you do decide to buy a mattress cover it should completely cover the mattress. Remember, too, that you will need to have a special cover for the pillow case and also for the duvet. Avoid a padded fabric headboard, where house dust mites could live. Even these measures will not remove all the mites from the bedroom.

The issue of reducing house dust mite numbers in bedrooms is an important one, but it is not an easy task to carry out and, as we have discussed in the previous question, there is no guarantee that it will help.

**What sort of carpet is best for my child's bedroom?**

If your child's asthma is clearly related to allergy, then the choice of bedroom floor covering can be important. Hardwood or linoleum floors are probably better than carpet because they do not collect dust in the same way. If your child's asthma is triggered by virus infections or exercise, then the type of carpet in the bedroom will not make much difference to the asthma.

Whenever possible, all soft furnishings should be washed frequently as this will cut down the number of dust mites as well. If dust levels in carpets are reduced as far as possible, then dust levels in the air will also fall. Remember that it is allergen levels in the air that cause problems, rather than allergen levels in the carpet.

**I am told that the house dust mite likes soft toys. Is there anything I can do to reduce the number of mites on the toys?**

Soft toys do accumulate dust and house dust mites and some children have literally dozens of these toys in their bedroom and on their beds. This increases their exposure to the mites, so reducing the overall toy population may help. Preparations called acaricide sprays kill house dust mites very effectively but the fumes of the spray may themselves set off an asthma attack. The spray treatment is quite expensive and treatment needs to be repeated regularly. Research still needs to be carried out before we can recommend using these particular sprays.

There is one rather unusual, but cheap and effective way of reducing dust mite numbers in soft toys. House dust mites do not survive if it is very cold (or if it is very hot for that matter). If you put soft toys in the freezer for at least 6 hours every week, exposure to this very cold temperature helps to get kill the mites. Do remember to vacuum the toys after they have been in the freezer to remove as much dust as possible. Washing soft toys at a hot temperature of at least 55°C will also kill the mites, but may destroy the toy in the process!

## Complementary therapies

We are not fond of prescribing asthma medicines for the sake of it, but we do so because they are effective and have been shown to work in carefully controlled research studies. Any medicine has the potential to cause side effects and because of this we understand that many people wish to explore the possibilities of non-medicine treatments for their asthma (and especially for their children's asthma). However, the benefits of conventional asthma medicines nearly always outweigh the potential disadvantages from their side effects.

Our difficulty is that very few of the non-medicine treatments for asthma have been shown to be effective in scientific research studies. We worry about our asthma patients stopping treatments that we know work, in favour of treatments that might work.

Uncontrolled asthma can be serious. This is why we prefer other treatments, such as homeopathy, to be additional to, rather than instead of your usual asthma medicines. *Complementary therapy* (rather than alternative medicine) is a term that is used for these other types of treatments (see the **Glossary**). Sometimes they are effective and as a result your asthma improves. In this case, you may be able to gradually reduce your usual asthma treatment. Always discuss this with your asthma nurse or doctor first because, if you suddenly stop your usual asthma medicines, your asthma may go badly out of control and you could have an asthma attack.

Doctors are sometimes accused of being 'anti' complementary treatments for the sake of it. We are not, but there can be risks in addition to the one we have outlined above. One of our worries is that complementary remedies themselves sometimes cause unwanted side effects. Some of the ingredients in complementary medicines do have an effect on asthma and, in fact, many modern medicines have been developed from some of these treatments.

For example:

- The remedy, Ma Huang (ephedra) is used in Traditional Chinese Medicine and contains ephedrine (adrenaline), a medicine that was once used widely to treat asthma. This caused a lot of unwanted side effects.

- The Japanese traditional medical system, called Kanpo, also makes use of ephedra.

- The Indian and Pakistani traditional medicine systems use plants called Datura, which contain substances that are useful for treating asthma. The medicine that was developed from this plant is called atropine, which dries up secretions, but it may cause serious side effects if the dose is not carefully measured.

- Herbal remedies are not licensed nor are they checked for their safety, but there are proposals to change this in the UK. It is often difficult to get any information on their possible side effects. While we keep an open mind about most of these remedies, we do need convincing evidence that they work before considering them as first-line treatments for asthma. It is important to remember that herbal remedies have the potential for side effects; there are already some concerns that St John's Wort may reduce the effectiveness of *theophylline* medicines.

- Traditional Chinese Medicine uses a number of different ingredients, usually boiled in water. Homeopathy uses single herbs diluted so much that there is virtually no active ingredient in the final prescribed remedy. It has been difficult to test the effect of homeopathy on people with asthma, mainly because different practitioners vary in their use of treatments. There is no doubt that some people do improve on homeopathy, but it is very difficult to know what aspect of the treatment helped. It is possible that the detailed consultation, where the homeopath spends a lot of time with the patient, is itself helpful, and the benefit may be due to what is called a *placebo* effect.

At the moment, we believe that there are no complementary (alternative) treatments that are as effective as the conventional preventer and reliever asthma treatments (these are described later in this chapter). It is, however, important to use the lowest doses of these medicines that control asthma symptoms.

**Do you think that complementary medicine can help people with asthma?**

Yes, we do. However, there is little scientific evidence that these treatments are effective on their own. They can be of help for some people when used together with conventional medical treatments. It is better to view them as 'complementary', rather than alternative. The idea of treating the whole person, rather than the illness, is an important part of many complementary therapies, and one which we strongly support.

There are several complementary treatments available, but we want to stress that the use of any of them should be in addition to and not instead of the conventional medical treatment. There is no place for these treatments in the management of acute asthma attacks, which are potentially dangerous and life threatening.

**What complementary therapies are available?**

There are a number of different types of complementary therapies:

- acupuncture
- homeopathy
- hypnosis
- breathing exercises, e.g. yoga and Buteyko.

Unfortunately there is no good evidence to show that either acupuncture or homeopathy benefits people with asthma. We have a little more information about breathing exercises. The aim of breathing exercises is to reduce *hyperventilation* (another name for overbreathing which upsets the normal balance of our oxygen and carbon dioxide levels in the blood). Blowing tests do not show any improvement in lung function after carrying out these exercises; however, people do report that it improves their quality of life, which is encouraging. If you are thinking of trying some of the complementary breathing exercises for asthma, do talk to your asthma nurse or doctor about them and continue your usual asthma treatment.

Hypnosis may help by improving relaxation but there is a risk that, under these circumstances, important asthma symptoms may not be recognized. This may be dangerous and, if you try hypnosis, we advise you to use your peak flow meter regularly to help identify whether your asthma is remaining under control. There is no sound evidence for using hypnosis in the treatment of asthma.

There is no scientific evidence either that naturopathy, aromatherapy or reflexology is of help to people with asthma. The methods of hair analysis and iridology for diagnosing allergy and asthma are unreliable and are often misleading.

If you are hoping to try any complementary treatments, do talk to your doctor or asthma nurse first and continue to take your usual asthma treatment. If you find that you obtain benefit from complementary treatments and are considering reducing your conventional asthma medicines, go and talk to your doctor or asthma nurse first so that you can plan how to do this safely.

### Does homeopathic treatment help asthma or make it worse?

It is usual to test treatments that claim to be of benefit, by doing clinical trials. These are research studies that compare the treatment in a number of people. The research is done by giving the test medicine (the one claimed to help) to some, while another group is given a 'dummy' medicine, called a placebo. The placebo medicine is made up to look and taste the same as the one being tested. Ideally, these studies are done in such a way that neither the doctor nor the people taking part know if they are using the placebo or the real medicine.

Homeopathy has been tested scientifically in this way more often than many other complementary therapies and none of the trials has shown that homeopathy is any more helpful than placebo in asthma. On the other hand there is certainly no evidence to suggest that it makes asthma worse. If the usual asthma treatment is stopped when the homeopathic treatment is started, asthma control may deteriorate, and this is why we strongly advise that your usual asthma treatments are continued.

Research has shown that homeopathy may help people with hay fever, but in the case of asthma the situation remains unclear, and there is not enough good scientific evidence for homeopathy to be recommended by us.

### Are breathing exercises and relaxation beneficial? If so, why are they never recommended by doctors?

Nowadays most doctors feel there is a place for breathing exercises for people with asthma. Generally, they are most useful for those people with the most severe asthma. During an asthma attack the muscles around the airways tighten; the most important thing is to get these muscles to relax, which will help to open up the airways. We have no conscious control over these muscles, and the best way to relax them quickly is by giving reliever asthma treatment. Fortunately, this is usually very effective and works quickly.

General relaxation exercises and controlled breathing can be extremely helpful. When an asthma attack begins, it is easy to become distressed and to overbreathe (hyperventilate). In the panic of an attack, breathing becomes rapid and shallow. This can irritate the airways and actually make matters worse. It is very helpful to learn how to breathe in a slow, relaxed way to prevent it from happening. If this does happen to you, you should practise these breathing exercises between attacks, when you are free of symptoms.

## *Medicines*

This section deals with the main medical treatments for asthma available in the UK.

There are many medicines available to treat asthma in the UK.

If your own treatment is not named in the book, it does not mean that you are receiving an unacceptable medicine, just that for reasons of space we cannot include all possible medicine names in the answer to each question. An added complication is that each medicine has a minimum of two names! The *generic name* is the basic, or real medicine name, but each medicine also has a *brand name*, given by the manufacturer. For example, the most frequently prescribed medicine for asthma is salbutamol (generic name). This is best known by the brand name Ventolin, used by its leading manufacturer, but also by other names such as Salamol, Airomir or Asmasal when marketed by a different company. We will refer to both brand and generic names, because many medicines are being prescribed by their generic names.

At present, inhaled asthma medicines are placed into one of two categories – preventers and relievers. Relievers are either short- or long-acting.

- **Preventer or *anti-inflammatory drugs*** prevent asthma symptoms if they are taken regularly. They are usually taken by the inhaled route. Steroid medicines are the most effective type of preventers. There are many different steroid inhalers (such as AeroBec, Alvesco, Asmanex, Becotide, Filair, Flixotide, and Pulmicort and Qvar). Other anti-inflammatory drugs are available (for example, Intal or Tilade) but are less effective than inhaled steroids.

- **Short-acting reliever medicines**, as the name suggests, relieve symptoms when they occur and therefore do not need to be taken regularly. They work within minutes and reach maximum benefit after 15–20 minutes. There is some evidence to suggest that they are more effective when they are taken occasionally rather than regularly.

- ***Long-acting reliever medicines*** are recommended for people who *are already taking preventer medicines but need additional treatment* to control their asthma symptoms. These reliever medicines, such as Serevent (salmeterol), Oxis (formoterol) and Foradil (formoterol), work for up to 12 hours, compared to the 4 hours for

short-acting relievers. All relievers work in the same way –
by relaxing tight muscles in the lining of the airways.

Other medicines include the following:

- *Leukotriene receptor antagonists* (LRTAs). These are
  available as tablets for children aged 2 and over and as
  granules for children as young as 6 months old. They work
  as preventer medicines but are not effective for all people
  with asthma. They are given as additional treatment to
  inhaled steroid and long-acting reliever inhalers, if asthma
  symptoms persist. They can also be used to treat rhinitis
  (inflammation of the nasal passages, e.g. hay fever) in older
  children and adults who are taking inhaled steroids for
  their asthma.

- **Combination treatments**. Symbicort is a combination
  asthma treatment which consists of an inhaled steroid
  preventer medicine, budesonide (Pulmicort) with a long-
  acting reliever medicine, formoterol (Oxis) in one inhaler.
  Seretide is a similar combination medicine but contains
  fluticasone (Flixotide) and salmeterol (Serevent). Seretide
  and Symbicort inhalers are prescribed frequently because
  many people find it is more convenient to take one inhaler
  device than two separate ones, and there is only one
  prescription charge if you have to pay.

## General

### Why does my daughter get free prescriptions for asthma in Wales but not in England?

The Welsh healthcare system is separate from the English and has
decided that asthma medicines should be free to all. In England,
unless you are exempt from charges, you must pay for asthma
prescriptions, as you know. We believe asthma medicines should
be available free of charge to all who need them, wherever they
live. It is not the only unusual or unjust case. In England, even

people with cystic fibrosis are not able to have free prescriptions, even though this is a serious and life-limiting chest disease.

### Do I have to use my preventer inhaler all the time, even when I am well?

This is an important question, and one that is frequently asked. After all it may be hard to accept that you should take treatment all the time if you have no symptoms. Firstly, we need to remember that the aim of modern asthma management is for you to be free from symptoms all the time, and to be able to lead a full life with no restrictions. Your preventer inhaler has been prescribed with that purpose in mind. It works by damping down, and controlling the swelling and mucus in your airways. This keeps your asthma symptoms to a minimum – as long as it is taken regularly. Even in mild asthma, inflammation is present in the airways of the lungs and, if left untreated, can cause long-term damage. If you stop taking the preventive treatment as soon as you are well, the symptoms are likely to return. If you have been free of symptoms for months, you may well be able to reduce the treatment gradually or stop it, but this should only be done after discussion with your doctor or asthma nurse.

### How often do I need to take my inhaler?

You should use your reliever inhalers, for example Ventolin Evohaler (salbutamol) or Bricanyl (terbutaline), whenever necessary. 'Whenever necessary' means when you have symptoms such as cough, wheeze or shortness of breath. These medicines are very important and can be life saving. These reliever medicines work quickly, and their effect should last for at least 4 hours. **If your reliever medicine does not work quickly, or its effects last for less than 4 hours, your asthma is uncontrolled and medical help is needed. Take extra reliever while you are waiting for help and advice.**

In severe attacks, reliever inhalers are used in high doses, that is 10–20 puffs (or more by injection or nebulizer).

Your preventer medicine needs to be taken regularly to work properly, even if you have no symptoms. There are two groups of preventer medicines:

- **Inhaled steroids** (AeroBec, Becotide, Becloforte, beclometasone, budesonide, Filair, Pulvinal [beclometasone], Qvar [beclometasone], Flixotide [fluticasone], and Pulmicort [budesonide]) work for about 12 hours, so they should be taken twice a day. Alvesco (ciclesonide) is a once-daily steroid, while Asmanex (mometasone) and budesonide can be used once or twice a day as well.

- **Intal** (sodium cromoglicate) is taken three to four times a day, although it is no longer used as a first-line preventer medicine. It may be helpful for the prevention of exercise symptoms if taken before exercise. **Tilade** (nedocromil sodium) is used two to four times a day. Both of these medicines are used less frequently now, as other asthma medicines are considered to be more effective.

### What is the difference between Pulmicort and Bricanyl?

Pulmicort is an inhaled steroid, a preventer medicine, while Bricanyl is a short-acting inhaled reliever treatment for asthma.

AeroBec, Becotide, Becloforte, beclometasone, budesonide, Filair, Pulvinal, Qvar (beclometasone), Flixotide (fluticasone), Alvesco (ciclesonide), Asmanex (mometasone) and Pulmicort (budesonide) are all inhaled steroids. They are anti-inflammatory drugs that help to prevent asthma attacks. They should be used regularly, twice a day, even if there are no symptoms. They are preventer medicines. The dose should be increased according to an agreed action plan for self-management, if symptoms are worsening or more relief medicine than usual is needed.

Bricanyl (terbutaline) and Ventolin (salbutamol) open up the tightened airways and are used only when symptoms happen. They are called reliever medicines. They should work quickly and you should feel better within 15 minutes. They usually work for at least 4 hours.

If your reliever medicine does not work quickly, or its effects last for less than 4 hours, your asthma is uncontrolled and medical help is needed. Take extra reliever while waiting for help or advice. These facts are important and can help you recognize when an attack is going to happen.

### I only cough at night, so why do I need my preventer inhaler during the day?

Taking your preventer every day will help to control your asthma even though you may be symptom free. When your asthma is mild, then symptoms such as cough may occur only on some days or nights. Your asthma is a condition that is present most of the time, even if it is not causing you any symptoms. There is a continuing inflammation (soreness) in the lining of your lungs, something like a slow burning fire where the embers are smouldering constantly and which burst into flames from time to time. This inflammation causes the walls of your airways to swell, and causes phlegm (consisting of cells and mucus) to collect on them. It can vary at different times, from being very mild to severe. When the inflammation flares up and becomes more severe, your symptoms will be present most of the day and night.

### Ventolin works better for me than Becotide, so why have I been prescribed Becotide?

Ventolin and Becotide work in different ways. Ventolin is a *bronchodilator*, which means that it 'dilates' or opens up the airways. Because of this, it relieves asthma symptoms quickly (and is therefore called a reliever). This is why you may feel, understandably, that this must be the best treatment. Becotide is an inhaled steroid and is purely a preventive treatment (a 'preventer'). It doesn't have an immediate effect on symptoms and needs to be taken twice a day to prevent asthma symptoms from occurring. It can sometimes take about a week before it starts to work, so many people feel, like you, that it 'works' less well than a reliever.

Inhaled steroids control the underlying inflammation of the airways. We do not know **exactly** how they work, but we do know that, taken on a long-term basis, they are highly effective. Most people find that once they take inhaled steroids regularly, their asthma symptoms get better, and they have less need to use their 'reliever' inhaler.

A word of caution though! The inhaled steroid is not a cure but it will keep your asthma under control. Forgetting to use your Becotide is how your asthma begins to get out of control again.

### If I forget to take my preventer inhaler one day, should I take twice the amount the next?

We appreciate that it is extremely easy to forget to take your preventer inhaler – particularly when you are well, and free from symptoms. It is of course much better if you can remember. There is usually no benefit from taking the doses you have missed although, if you are having asthma symptoms, it may be worth taking extra inhaled steroid medicine. If you do have symptoms, we would advise you to increase the dose of your preventer four or five times; this applies to most preventers, though we suggest you ask your doctor or asthma nurse to put clear details on your action plan.

### What does 'when necessary' mean for my Bricanyl?

'When necessary' means when you have symptoms, such as cough, wheeze, chest tightness or shortness of breath. Bricanyl and Ventolin are the two reliever medicines used most frequently in the UK. Your Bricanyl can be used intermittently when you get symptoms, rather than regularly. Many doctors believe that it is more effective when it is used in this way.

However, if your asthma is severe or chronic, 'when necessary' is usually in addition to your regular doses of reliever inhaler medicine.

### What should I use first – reliever or preventer inhaler?

Until fairly recently, the standard advice would have been: 'always use your reliever before your preventer', because the reliever should open up the airways enough to let the preventer get deeper into your lungs. However, it takes 15–20 minutes before you get maximum benefit from the reliever inhaler, so this advice is not very logical! If you need to take regular reliever treatment, if you always take it in the same order, for example blue before brown, it will help you to remember which inhalers you have already used.

Currently many people do not take their reliever on a regular basis, only if they have symptoms. They may also take it before exercise to stop symptoms developing. If your asthma is well controlled, and you have no symptoms, then the airways are fully open, and it really isn't necessary to take your reliever. Just take the preventer on its own!

**I try to avoid taking my Ventolin if I feel I have been using it frequently. Does this do me more harm than actually taking it?**

Yes it does, because it is not wise to ignore asthma symptoms. If you need to take extra Ventolin your asthma is not under control. However, you should take it if you have troublesome asthma symptoms. You may need other asthma medicines or even a short course of steroid tablets to gain quick control of your asthma. Speak with your doctor or asthma nurse as soon as you can. You need to have an assessment of your asthma to see if it can be better controlled. It is possible that some changes are needed to your treatment.

**What is the difference between Beconase and Becotide?**

Becotide is used to treat asthma and Beconase is used for rhinitis, which is a similar condition to asthma affecting the lining of the nose. Rhinitis, like asthma, is often triggered by an allergy, and can occur all the year round. Hay fever is the most common form of allergic rhinitis, and its medical name is seasonal rhinitis.

Rhinitis can spark off an asthma attack, so it is important to take your treatment regularly if rhinitis flares up. In seasonal rhinitis (hay fever), it is really best to start the preventer medicine just before you anticipate your symptoms, for example when the pollen counts are reported to be rising early in summer. There are a number of medicines that are used to treat both the nose and the chest.

There are a number of inhaled steroid preventer medicines that can be used for nose symptoms (allergic rhinitis or hay fever) as well as for the chest (asthma). Many of the same medicines are used for both asthma and rhinitis. For example:

- Asmanex (mometasone) is available as an inhaler as well as a once-daily nasal spray (Nasonex).

- Becotide (beclometasone) is available as an inhaler as well as a nasal spray (Beconase).

- Flixotide (fluticasone) is available as an inhaler as well as a once-daily nasal spray (Flixonase).

- Pulmicort (budesonide) is available as an inhaler as well as a twice-daily nasal spray (Rhinocort).

Many people with asthma may find themselves using both an inhaled steroid and a nasal steroid, such as Becotide plus Beconase. Usually this will be because of allergic rhinitis but less commonly because they have polyps in the nose. These polyps are fleshy swellings of the nasal lining. They are not cancerous, and usually they do shrink and respond very well to nasal steroid treatment.

**I am using a steroid inhaler for my asthma, a steroid nose spray for hay fever as well as a steroid cream for my eczema. Is this all right?**

Yes it is, but the lowest necessary dose of steroid medicines should always be used. If your asthma is under good control, it is possible that the dose could be reduced, but not so low that you start to get asthma symptoms. If your eczema is under control you may need minimal or no steroid cream. You do need to continue to use plenty of emollient (moisturizing) creams to stop your skin becoming dry and sore. If your nose symptoms are better after the hay fever season, you probably don't need to continue to take your nose spray all the year round. Speak with your asthma nurse or doctor to see how your medicines can be reduced without your asthma or nose symptoms becoming worse or your eczema flaring up.

**If Pulmicort keeps my asthma under control, can it work on its own without Bricanyl?**

Yes it can, and increasingly we are suggesting that this is the way in which treatment should be taken – using Pulmicort (or another preventer) regularly, and reserving reliever treatments for when symptoms occur. In fact a test of how well controlled your asthma is, is to ask how often you have needed to use your Bricanyl. If it is well controlled (and you can tell this by charting your peak flow and noting your symptoms – see Chapter 3), Pulmicort can maintain very good control without the need to use your Bricanyl, although it should always be available just in case your asthma flares up.

Please remember that, however well controlled your asthma seems to be, it is a variable condition, and can change rapidly because of a sudden exposure to trigger factors (see Chapter 2).

**What exactly does prednisolone do?**

Prednisolone is one of a group of medicines whose proper name is *corticosteroids*. We do not completely understand all of its actions in treating asthma. However, we do know that it reduces and dampens down inflammation dramatically and controls the production of phlegm.

Prednisolone is the most commonly prescribed *oral steroid* medicine in the UK. It is used to treat acute attacks of asthma and, less commonly, as long-term therapy for chronic severe asthma. In acute asthma, it is important to make sure that high enough doses are prescribed, and that it is given for a long enough time for the inflammation to subside. In an adult such a dose would usually be in the range of 30–60 mg/day, and for a child 10–40 mg/day. It works better when the tablets are taken all together in one dose (usually after breakfast) rather than in divided doses through the day.

There is a soluble form of prednisolone that dissolves in water. This is extremely useful for children, and for people who find tablets hard to swallow. Prednisolone can also be given in a special coated form to reduce the risks of indigestion and upset to the stomach, which otherwise can be troublesome side effects. Taking the tablets with food, rather than on an empty stomach, also reduces the risk of indigestion.

**My doctor says that I would need to use my reliever inhaler much less if I started using another inhaler called salmeterol, as well as my preventer. What is salmeterol, and why is it different?**

Salmeterol (brand name Serevent) is a long-acting inhaled medicine belonging to the group of medicines called *beta agonist* bronchodilators (see the ***Glossary*** for more details of this group of medicines). Formoterol (brand name Foradil and Oxis) is a similar medicine and is used as an alternative. These medicines are related to the short-acting reliever treatments (such as Ventolin and Bricanyl) with which we are familiar, but differ in that they keep the airways open for longer, lasting for about 12 hours. They are usually taken twice a day and are not intended for immediate relief of symptoms. Serevent comes in either a standard pressurized inhaler, a Diskhaler, or an Accuhaler. Foradil comes as a dry powder capsule for use in a *breath-activated inhaler* and Oxis in a Turbohaler *dry powder device*. The effect is noticeable after 3–10 minutes, but the full benefit is not generally noticed until after several doses of the medicine. Because of its long-lasting action, it can be particularly useful in treating people who have night-time symptoms.

Like preventers, these medicines should be taken regularly to gain full benefit. Salmeterol and formoterol are not a replacement for, or an alternative to, inhaled steroids or any other preventive asthma treatments. They form an **additional treatment to the usual dose of preventer medicine**, if these do not control asthma symptoms, rather than being a first-line treatment. These medicines should always be used together with steroid inhaler medicine. It is very important that inhaled steroids or other preventive treatments are not stopped when salmeterol or formoterol is prescribed. Many people notice that they need little, or none, of their short-acting relieving treatment once they start taking one of these long-acting bronchodilators.

**What is ciclosporin? I have heard of it in relation to asthma so why are we not using it as a treatment yet?**

Ciclosporin is a very powerful and expensive medicine that works by reducing the body's response to inflammation. It is used to treat people with a number of diseases such as cancer, or who have had transplants. It is an 'immunosuppressive' medicine, because it dampens down (suppresses) the body's immune system, which protects it against infections.

Ciclosporin is sometimes used to treat people with very severe asthma because it works against inflammatory changes within the lungs. It is used only if asthma cannot be controlled by other usual asthma medicines. Methotrexate is another powerful medicine with anti-inflammatory effects, which is also used to treat severe asthma.

Both of these medicines have potentially severe side effects, which make them unsuitable for treating mild or moderate asthma. For ciclosporin, apart from suppressing the body's own immune system (which can lead to severe infections), these side effects include anaemia, kidney damage, rashes and severe overgrowth of body hair. Even though ciclosporin seems to be very effective, it is too toxic to recommend for routine use. It is only prescribed initially by a respiratory specialist doctor.

**Why won't my GP prescribe antibiotics for me to have at home so that I can take them at the first sign of a chest infection? This form of treatment means less time off work for me, and less pressure from my employers. This pressure tends to make my asthma worse.**

This is a rather tricky question, which, without knowing your individual details, we will have to answer in general terms. The difficulty arises in having to distinguish between asthma and a true chest infection. Although antibiotics may help to clear a chest infection rapidly, they are not often helpful in the treatment of asthma. Although asthma is often triggered by an infection, such as the common cold, this infection is nearly always caused by a virus. Viruses are not affected at all by antibiotics, so there is no point giving them for the treatment of virus infections.

The symptoms of an asthma attack may resemble a chest infection, with coughing, wheezing and shortness of breath. Asthma may also cause you to cough up lots of phlegm – leading to the false impression that your symptoms are due to an infection that needs antibiotics. It is usually much better for you to increase your asthma medication at the start of these symptoms. If they do not improve, you need to consult your doctor or asthma nurse to see if any other treatment is needed.

### Are there particular times of the day when medication should be taken, or should I leave it as long as possible before taking it?

The answer to this depends on the medication you are taking. Inhaled steroids (such as AeroBec, Asmabec, Becloforte, beclometasone, Becotide, budesonide, Flixotide, Pulmicort, Pulvinal [beclometasone] and Qvar) are usually taken twice daily. The actual time does not matter, but they are usually taken every night and morning. If you take them before brushing your teeth, it becomes part of a routine, but also ensures that you rinse your mouth out afterwards. This reduces the chance of side effects, especially *thrush* in the throat. Asmanex is taken once or twice a day, while Alvesco is a once-daily treatment. Alvesco doesn't work until it gets into the lungs so local side effects are reduced. The benefit from preventer treatments comes from taking them regularly, and to do this it is best to have a routine.

Reliever treatments such as Ventolin, Aerolin, Asmasal, Airomir (salbutamol) or Bricanyl (terbutaline) should be taken when you feel wheezy or short of breath, or if you feel an attack coming on – there are no set times for these.

Serevent (salmeterol) and Foradil (formoterol) and Oxis (formoterol) belong to a class of bronchodilator treatments that have a long action of 10–12 hours. They should be taken regularly, twice daily.

You don't have to be so rigid in the times when you take your medication but the preventers and long-acting relievers do need to be taken twice a day to work properly. You need to work out when to take them so that they fit in with your lifestyle.

**Should I have an anti-flu injection?**

If you are prone to bad attacks of asthma during the winter months, the answer is yes.

Virus infections are important triggers for asthma in many people. Influenza (better known as 'flu) is a particularly important virus infection. It can cause serious pneumonia, particularly in elderly people or those with chronic chest trouble. For people with asthma, 'flu may bring on a severe episode of asthma. It is generally recommended that all these people should have protection against 'flu.

An anti-flu injection once a year will help to prevent the illness, or at least reduce its severity. There are few side effects from this injection. Some people are unlucky, and they suffer from a mild 'flu-like illness for a few days after the injection. Many general practices run 'flu clinics where the 'flu vaccine is available free of charge. If you have a prescription for your 'flu vaccine, you may have to pay a prescription charge if you are not eligible for free prescriptions. Those who are exempt from prescription charges do not pay in any case.

**I have asthma and eczema. I take my steroid inhaler twice each day, so why does my doctor tell me to be careful with the steroid cream for my eczema?**

We suspect your doctor is trying to ensure that you do not use too much steroid. Taking your steroid asthma medicines twice a day is an excellent way of helping to keep your asthma under control. Eczema and asthma often occur together but need to be treated separately. The most important treatment for eczema is to use plenty of moisturizing creams or ointments. These help to prevent the skin becoming dry and losing moisture. These creams or ointments are known as emollients. Emollients can be used whenever the skin feels dry and/or itchy. They should be used at least twice a day, but there is no limit as to how often they can be used. If you have eczema, it is sensible to avoid perfumed soaps and bath lotions and to avoid using biological washing powders. These may irritate your skin and make your eczema worse.

Steroid creams and ointments are kept to treat 'flare-ups' or severe eczema. There are different strengths available but, as in asthma, the lowest strength (dose) possible should be used. Once the eczema is under control, then the steroid skin treatment may be stopped or stepped down to a lower strength. Emollients should continue to be used even if your eczema is under control.

### Are there any long-term problems if I use a steroid inhaler for my asthma and steroid cream for my eczema?

For most people, using both steroid inhalers and steroid creams does not cause any problems. However, the total amount of steroid that you are exposed to is higher if two steroid medicines are used. Steroid medicines are potent, and as with any medicines, there is always the possibility and potential for side effects. Do not stop using your inhaler or your eczema medicine. Talk to your doctor or asthma nurse about your asthma and your eczema, in order to maximize the benefits, while minimizing the overall total dose.

### I sneeze a lot and my nose is blocked in the spring time. I can't believe this is hay fever as I thought this only happened in the summer?

Yes it can be hay fever. It is a term used for nose, throat and eye symptoms that happen as a result of an allergy to grass pollen in the summer. Grass pollens can cause 'hay fever' symptoms in June and July as a result of an allergic response to grass pollens. Tree pollens cause the same sort of nose and eye symptoms, but much earlier in the year. In fact tree pollens can start as early as February! The trees that cause the most problems are birch and hazel.

It sounds as if you are allergic to tree pollens. Speak with your asthma nurse, doctor or pharmacist because you may benefit from using a regular steroid nose spray as well as occasional antihistamines. If you start the steroid nose spray just before 'your' pollen season and continue to take it for as long as the pollen is around, you may find that your 'hay fever' symptoms are kept under control. More recently a tablet called montelukast (Singulair) has been given a licence for the treatment of rhinitis, so long as an individual has asthma, which is being treated with inhaled steroids as well. For some people, this treatment may be helpful.

**Is it all right to use eye drops as well as inhalers?**

It may seem strange but certain eye drops that are prescribed for the condition glaucoma may, in fact, aggravate asthma. Glaucoma is a common cause of blindness, which can be prevented with the right treatment. Timoptol is the most important of these medicines. It is a beta-blocker medicine, which means it has the opposite effect to the (beta-stimulant) action of the reliever inhalers. Even the tiny doses of these eye drops that are absorbed into the system have been known to have a bad effect on asthma. Most other types of eye drops used for glaucoma cause no problems. If you are unlucky enough to have both glaucoma and asthma, you should discuss this problem with your doctor or asthma nurse and alternative eye drop medicines can be prescribed.

## Devices

There are many different inhalers available which contain anti-asthma medicines. They can be divided into:

- metered dose inhalers
- breath-activated inhalers
- dry powder inhalers
- spacer devices
- nebulizers.

### Metered dose inhalers

These are sometimes called the 'press and breathe' inhalers. They use a special sort of gas which is harmless, to help release the

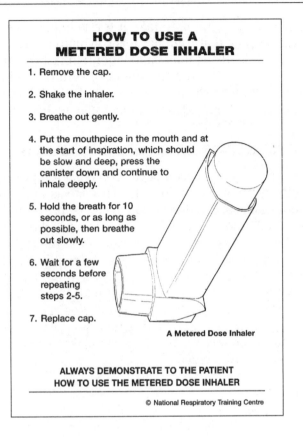

**Figure 4.1** How to use the metered dose inhaler.

medicine as a fine spray. You need to breathe in at exactly the same time as the canister is pressed down, but because the spray is released very quickly, it is not always easy to use. See Figure 4.1 on how to use the metered dose inhaler.

### Breath-activated devices

There are currently two breath-activated devices. These are:

- the Airomir Autohaler
- the Easi-Breathe.

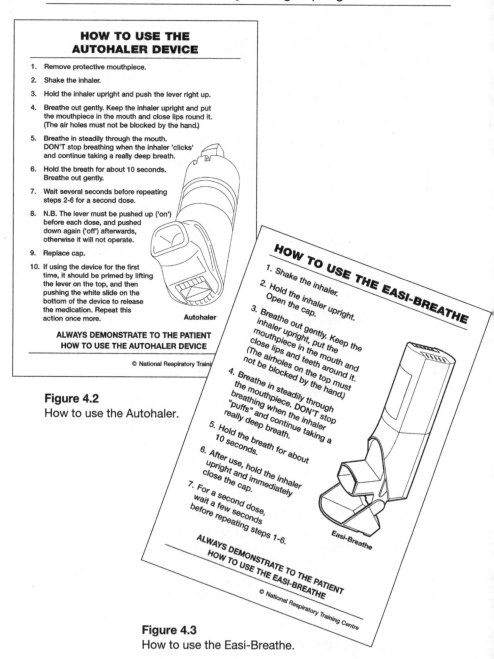

**HOW TO USE THE AUTOHALER DEVICE**

1. Remove protective mouthpiece.
2. Shake the inhaler.
3. Hold the inhaler upright and push the lever right up.
4. Breathe out gently. Keep the inhaler upright and put the mouthpiece in the mouth and close lips round it. (The air holes must not be blocked by the hand.)
5. Breathe in steadily through the mouth. DON'T stop breathing when the inhaler 'clicks' and continue taking a really deep breath.
6. Hold the breath for about 10 seconds. Breathe out gently.
7. Wait several seconds before repeating steps 2-6 for a second dose.
8. N.B. The lever must be pushed up ('on') before each dose, and pushed down again ('off') afterwards, otherwise it will not operate.
9. Replace cap.
10. If using the device for the first time, it should be primed by lifting the lever on the top, and then pushing the white slide on the bottom of the device to release the medication. Repeat this action once more.

ALWAYS DEMONSTRATE TO THE PATIENT HOW TO USE THE AUTOHALER DEVICE

© National Respiratory Training

**Figure 4.2**
How to use the Autohaler.

**HOW TO USE THE EASI-BREATHE**

1. Shake the inhaler.
2. Hold the inhaler upright. Open the cap.
3. Breathe out gently. Keep the inhaler upright, put the mouthpiece in the mouth and close lips and teeth around it. (The airholes on the top must not be blocked by the hand)
4. Breathe in steadily through the mouthpiece. DON'T stop breathing when the inhaler "puffs" and continue taking a really deep breath.
5. Hold the breath for about 10 seconds.
6. After use, hold the inhaler upright and immediately close the cap.
7. For a second dose, wait a few seconds before repeating steps 1-6.

ALWAYS DEMONSTRATE TO THE PATIENT HOW TO USE THE EASI-BREATHE

© National Respiratory Training Centre

**Figure 4.3**
How to use the Easi-Breathe.

The medicine is contained in canisters (like the metered dose inhaler) but the dose of medicine is not released until you breathe in. These devices are easier to use than the metered dose inhaler because they do not rely on good hand–breath coordination. See Figures 4.2 and 4.3 on how to use these devices.

## Dry powder inhalers

These can be divided into single-dose or reservoir devices.

### Single-dose dry powder inhalers, e.g. Accuhaler, Aerolizer, Diskhaler

- The **Accuhaler** contains 60 doses of medicine in an enclosed foil strip within the inhaler. Each dose is separately sealed and is not exposed until the lever is set (see Figure 4.4).

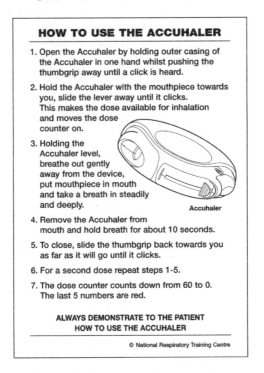

**HOW TO USE THE ACCUHALER**

1. Open the Accuhaler by holding outer casing of the Accuhaler in one hand whilst pushing the thumbgrip away until a click is heard.

2. Hold the Accuhaler with the mouthpiece towards you, slide the lever away until it clicks. This makes the dose available for inhalation and moves the dose counter on.

3. Holding the Accuhaler level, breathe out gently away from the device, put mouthpiece in mouth and take a breath in steadily and deeply.

   Accuhaler

4. Remove the Accuhaler from mouth and hold breath for about 10 seconds.

5. To close, slide the thumbgrip back towards you as far as it will go until it clicks.

6. For a second dose repeat steps 1-5.

7. The dose counter counts down from 60 to 0. The last 5 numbers are red.

ALWAYS DEMONSTRATE TO THE PATIENT
HOW TO USE THE ACCUHALER

© National Respiratory Training Centre

**Figure 4.4** How to use the Accuhaler.

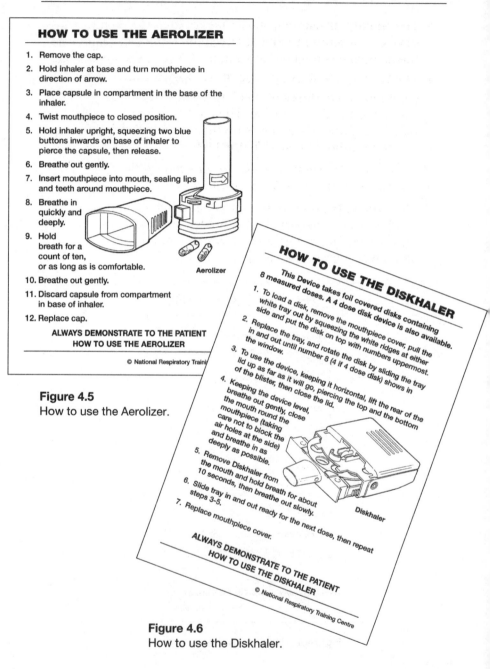

**HOW TO USE THE AEROLIZER**

1. Remove the cap.
2. Hold inhaler at base and turn mouthpiece in direction of arrow.
3. Place capsule in compartment in the base of the inhaler.
4. Twist mouthpiece to closed position.
5. Hold inhaler upright, squeezing two blue buttons inwards on base of inhaler to pierce the capsule, then release.
6. Breathe out gently.
7. Insert mouthpiece into mouth, sealing lips and teeth around mouthpiece.
8. Breathe in quickly and deeply.
9. Hold breath for a count of ten, or as long as is comfortable.
10. Breathe out gently.
11. Discard capsule from compartment in base of inhaler.
12. Replace cap.

**ALWAYS DEMONSTRATE TO THE PATIENT HOW TO USE THE AEROLIZER**

© National Respiratory Traini

**Figure 4.5**
How to use the Aerolizer.

**HOW TO USE THE DISKHALER**

This Device takes foil covered disks containing 8 measured doses. A 4 dose disk device is also available.

1. To load a disk, remove the mouthpiece cover, pull the white tray out by squeezing the white ridges at either side and put the disk on top with numbers uppermost.
2. Replace the tray, and rotate the disk by sliding the tray in and out until number 8 (4 if 4 dose disk) shows in the window.
3. To use the device, keeping it horizontal, lift the rear of the lid up as far as it will go, piercing the top and the bottom of the blister, then close the lid.
4. Keeping the device level, breathe out gently, close the mouth round the mouthpiece (taking care not to block the air holes at the side) and breathe in as deeply as possible.
5. Remove Diskhaler from the mouth and hold breath for about 10 seconds, then breathe out slowly.
6. Slide tray in and out ready for the next dose, then repeat steps 3-5.
7. Replace mouthpiece cover.

**ALWAYS DEMONSTRATE TO THE PATIENT HOW TO USE THE DISKHALER**

© National Respiratory Training Centre

**Figure 4.6**
How to use the Diskhaler.

- The **Aerolizer** uses capsules that are loaded into the device. Holes are pricked at each end of the capsule before the medicine is inhaled (see Figure 4.5).

- The **Diskhaler** has foil disks that contain either four or eight individual doses of medicine. These disks are placed inside the Diskhaler device. The medicine is released by puncturing one of the doses on the disk which then allows you to breathe it in (see Figure 4.6).

*Reservoir dry powder devices, e.g. Easyhaler, Clickhaler, Novolizer, Pulvinal, Turbohaler and Twisthaler*

- The **Easyhaler** device is compact and releases one dose of medicine, each time the top is pressed down. It has a numerical counter and a see-through window where the amount of powder can be seen (see Figure 4.7).

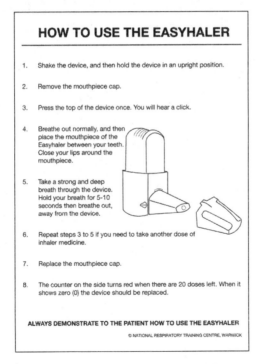

**HOW TO USE THE EASYHALER**

1. Shake the device, and then hold the device in an upright position.

2. Remove the mouthpiece cap.

3. Press the top of the device once. You will hear a click.

4. Breathe out normally, and then place the mouthpiece of the Easyhaler between your teeth. Close your lips around the mouthpiece.

5. Take a strong and deep breath through the device. Hold your breath for 5-10 seconds then breathe out, away from the device.

6. Repeat steps 3 to 5 if you need to take another dose of inhaler medicine.

7. Replace the mouthpiece cap.

8. The counter on the side turns red when there are 20 doses left. When it shows zero (0) the device should be replaced.

ALWAYS DEMONSTRATE TO THE PATIENT HOW TO USE THE EASYHALER

© NATIONAL RESPIRATORY TRAINING CENTRE, WARWICK

**Figure 4.7** How to use the Easyhaler.

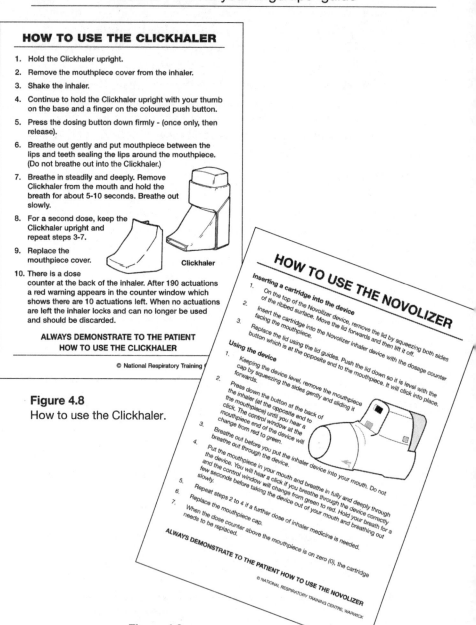

## HOW TO USE THE CLICKHALER

1. Hold the Clickhaler upright.
2. Remove the mouthpiece cover from the inhaler.
3. Shake the inhaler.
4. Continue to hold the Clickhaler upright with your thumb on the base and a finger on the coloured push button.
5. Press the dosing button down firmly - (once only, then release).
6. Breathe out gently and put mouthpiece between the lips and teeth sealing the lips around the mouthpiece. (Do not breathe out into the Clickhaler.)
7. Breathe in steadily and deeply. Remove Clickhaler from the mouth and hold the breath for about 5-10 seconds. Breathe out slowly.
8. For a second dose, keep the Clickhaler upright and repeat steps 3-7.
9. Replace the mouthpiece cover.
10. There is a dose counter at the back of the inhaler. After 190 actuations a red warning appears in the counter window which shows there are 10 actuations left. When no actuations are left the inhaler locks and can no longer be used and should be discarded.

Clickhaler

**ALWAYS DEMONSTRATE TO THE PATIENT HOW TO USE THE CLICKHALER**

© National Respiratory Training

### Figure 4.8
How to use the Clickhaler.

## HOW TO USE THE NOVOLIZER

### Inserting a cartridge into the device

1. On the top of the Novolizer device, remove the lid by squeezing both sides of the ribbed surface. Move the lid forwards and then lift it off.
2. Insert the cartridge into the Novolizer inhaler device with the dosage counter facing the mouthpiece.
3. Replace the lid using the lid guides. Push the lid down so it is level with the button which is at the opposite end to the mouthpiece. It will click into place.

### Using the device

1. Keeping the device level, remove the mouthpiece cap by squeezing the sides gently and sliding it forwards.
2. Press down the button at the back of the inhaler (at the opposite end to the mouthpiece) until you hear a click. The control window at the mouthpiece end of the device will change from red to green.
3. Breathe out before you put the inhaler device into your mouth. Do not breathe out through the device.
4. Put the mouthpiece in your mouth and breathe in fully and deeply through the device. You will hear a click if you breathe through the device correctly and the control window will change from green to red. Hold your breath for a few seconds before taking the device out of your mouth and breathing out slowly.
5. Repeat steps 2 to 4 if a further dose of inhaler medicine is needed.
6. Replace the mouthpiece cap.
7. When the dose counter above the mouthpiece is on zero (0), the cartridge needs to be replaced.

**ALWAYS DEMONSTRATE TO THE PATIENT HOW TO USE THE NOVOLIZER**

© NATIONAL RESPIRATORY TRAINING CENTRE, WARWICK

### Figure 4.9
How to use the Novolizer.

- The **Clickhaler** has a numerical counter and looks a little like a metered dose inhaler. When the top is pressed to activate one dose, a clicking sound is heard – hence the name of the device. The slightly elongated mouthpiece is ideal for children who have fixed braces on their teeth because they are able to seal their lips securely around the mouthpiece before breathing in the medicine (see Figure 4.8).

- The **Novolizer** is a novel device with a replaceable medication cartridge. There is a numerical counter as well as a small window that changes from green to red following correct inhalation technique (see Figure 4.9).

- The **Pulvinal** device releases one dose at a time when you twist the body of the inhaler. This device has a see-through

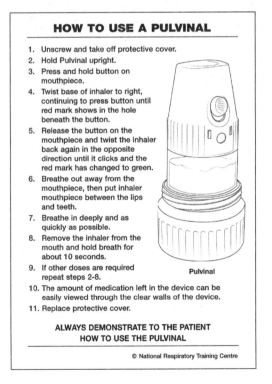

**HOW TO USE A PULVINAL**

1. Unscrew and take off protective cover.
2. Hold Pulvinal upright.
3. Press and hold button on mouthpiece.
4. Twist base of inhaler to right, continuing to press button until red mark shows in the hole beneath the button.
5. Release the button on the mouthpiece and twist the inhaler back again in the opposite direction until it clicks and the red mark has changed to green.
6. Breathe out away from the mouthpiece, then put inhaler mouthpiece between the lips and teeth.
7. Breathe in deeply and as quickly as possible.
8. Remove the inhaler from the mouth and hold breath for about 10 seconds.
9. If other doses are required repeat steps 2-8.
10. The amount of medication left in the device can be easily viewed through the clear walls of the device.
11. Replace protective cover.

Pulvinal

**ALWAYS DEMONSTRATE TO THE PATIENT HOW TO USE THE PULVINAL**

© National Respiratory Training Centre

**Figure 4.10** How to use the Pulvinal.

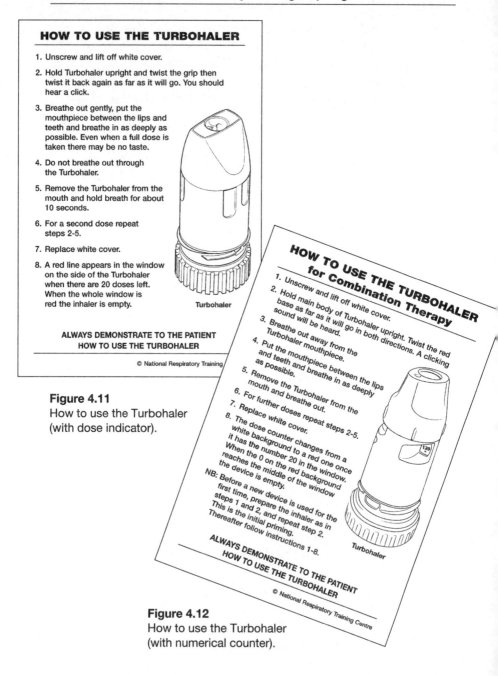

## HOW TO USE THE TURBOHALER

1. Unscrew and lift off white cover.

2. Hold Turbohaler upright and twist the grip then twist it back again as far as it will go. You should hear a click.

3. Breathe out gently, put the mouthpiece between the lips and teeth and breathe in as deeply as possible. Even when a full dose is taken there may be no taste.

4. Do not breathe out through the Turbohaler.

5. Remove the Turbohaler from the mouth and hold breath for about 10 seconds.

6. For a second dose repeat steps 2-5.

7. Replace white cover.

8. A red line appears in the window on the side of the Turbohaler when there are 20 doses left. When the whole window is red the inhaler is empty.

Turbohaler

**ALWAYS DEMONSTRATE TO THE PATIENT
HOW TO USE THE TURBOHALER**

© National Respiratory Training

**Figure 4.11**
How to use the Turbohaler
(with dose indicator).

## HOW TO USE THE TURBOHALER
### for Combination Therapy

1. Unscrew and lift off white cover.

2. Hold main body of Turbohaler upright. Twist the red base as far as it will go in both directions. A clicking sound will be heard.

3. Breathe out away from the Turbohaler mouthpiece.

4. Put the mouthpiece between the lips and teeth and breathe in as deeply as possible.

5. Remove the Turbohaler from the mouth and breathe out.

6. For further doses repeat steps 2-5.

7. Replace white cover.

8. The dose counter changes from a white background to a red one once it has the number 20 in the window. When the 0 on the red background reaches the middle of the window the device is empty.

NB: Before a new device is used for the first time, prepare the inhaler as in steps 1 and 2, and repeat step 2. This is the initial priming. Thereafter follow instructions 1-8.

**ALWAYS DEMONSTRATE TO THE PATIENT
HOW TO USE THE TURBOHALER**

© National Respiratory Training Centre

Turbohaler

**Figure 4.12**
How to use the Turbohaler
(with numerical counter).

body so that you can check how much medicine is left (see Figure 4.10).

- The **Turbohaler** also releases one dose at a time if the base is twisted. It contains either an indicator or a numbered counter, which helps you to check how much medicine is left (see Figures 4.11 and 4.12).

- The **Twisthaler** device releases the medicine ready to breathe in when you take the inhaler top off. It also has a numbered counter, which locks once the last dose is used and prevents the inhaler device being used again (see Figure 4.13).

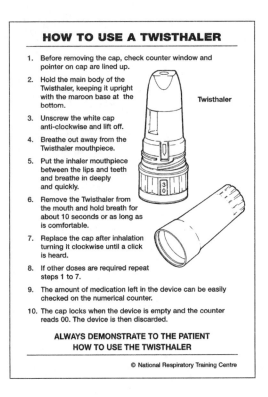

### HOW TO USE A TWISTHALER

1. Before removing the cap, check counter window and pointer on cap are lined up.

2. Hold the main body of the Twisthaler, keeping it upright with the maroon base at the bottom.

3. Unscrew the white cap anti-clockwise and lift off.

4. Breathe out away from the Twisthaler mouthpiece.

5. Put the inhaler mouthpiece between the lips and teeth and breathe in deeply and quickly.

6. Remove the Twisthaler from the mouth and hold breath for about 10 seconds or as long as is comfortable.

7. Replace the cap after inhalation turning it clockwise until a click is heard.

8. If other doses are required repeat steps 1 to 7.

9. The amount of medication left in the device can be easily checked on the numerical counter.

10. The cap locks when the device is empty and the counter reads 00. The device is then discarded.

**ALWAYS DEMONSTRATE TO THE PATIENT HOW TO USE THE TWISTHALER**

© National Respiratory Training Centre

**Figure 4.13** How to use the Twisthaler.

**Now that CFCs are being phased out, what will happen to asthma inhalers?**

You are quite right; CFC inhalers are being phased out. In order to protect the earth's atmosphere, the substances (CFC *propellants*) that provide the energy for the pressurized asthma inhalers are being phased out. The replacement propellant is hydrofluoralkane or HFA. All salbutamol inhalers now use HFA propellants but at the moment there is only one beclometasone HFA inhaler – Qvar. Qvar must be prescribed by its brand or trade name rather than the 'generic' name of beclometasone to make sure you always get the same inhaler medicine from the pharmacy. This is important because it is used at half the dose of the other CFC beclometasone products. The Qvar spray particles are much smaller than the CFC equivalent and it allows the spray to reach the small airways of the lungs more easily.

## Spacer devices

These holding chambers are used together with a metered dose inhaler. The inhaler is sprayed into the spacer, which traps the medicine. This allows enough time for the medicine to be inhaled by normal breathing through the spacer mouthpiece. Children under the age of about 3 years of age will need to use a face mask attached to the mouthpiece of the spacer device. These devices include:

- Large-volume spacers, e.g. Volumatic, Nebuhaler (see Figures 4.14, 4.15 and 4.16). The Volumatic is not being made any longer, although the spacer device is likely to be around for a number of years.

- Small-volume spacers, e.g. Nebuchamber, Aerochamber, Pocket Chamber, Able Spacer (see Figures 4.17, 4.18, 4.19, 4.20).

Face masks are available for both large- and small-volume spacers (see Figures 4.21, 4.22, 4.23 and 4.24).

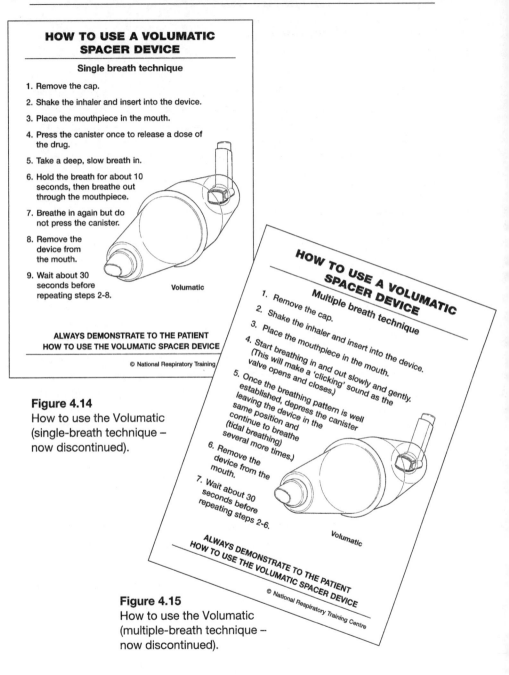

**HOW TO USE A VOLUMATIC SPACER DEVICE**

**Single breath technique**

1. Remove the cap.

2. Shake the inhaler and insert into the device.

3. Place the mouthpiece in the mouth.

4. Press the canister once to release a dose of the drug.

5. Take a deep, slow breath in.

6. Hold the breath for about 10 seconds, then breathe out through the mouthpiece.

7. Breathe in again but do not press the canister.

8. Remove the device from the mouth.

9. Wait about 30 seconds before repeating steps 2-8.

Volumatic

**ALWAYS DEMONSTRATE TO THE PATIENT HOW TO USE THE VOLUMATIC SPACER DEVICE**

© National Respiratory Training

**Figure 4.14**
How to use the Volumatic (single-breath technique – now discontinued).

**HOW TO USE A VOLUMATIC SPACER DEVICE**

**Multiple breath technique**

1. Remove the cap.

2. Shake the inhaler and insert into the device.

3. Place the mouthpiece in the mouth.

4. Start breathing in and out slowly and gently. (This will make a 'clicking' sound as the valve opens and closes.)

5. Once the breathing pattern is well established, depress the canister leaving the device in the same position and continue to breathe (tidal breathing) several more times.)

6. Remove the device from the mouth.

7. Wait about 30 seconds before repeating steps 2-6.

Volumatic

**ALWAYS DEMONSTRATE TO THE PATIENT HOW TO USE THE VOLUMATIC SPACER DEVICE**

© National Respiratory Training Centre

**Figure 4.15**
How to use the Volumatic (multiple-breath technique – now discontinued).

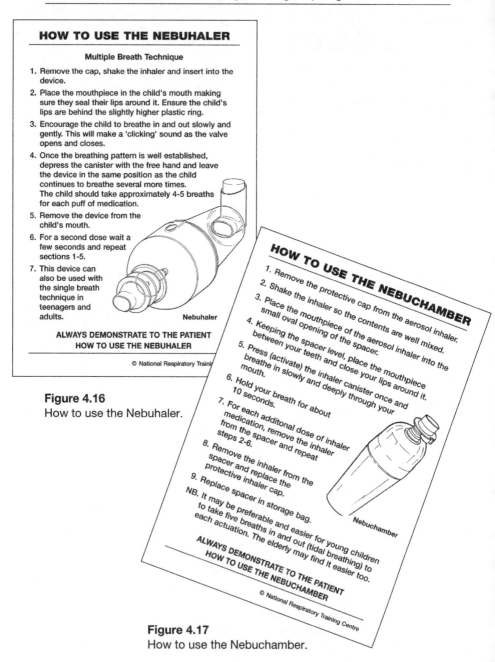

**HOW TO USE THE NEBUHALER**

**Multiple Breath Technique**

1. Remove the cap, shake the inhaler and insert into the device.

2. Place the mouthpiece in the child's mouth making sure they seal their lips around it. Ensure the child's lips are behind the slightly higher plastic ring.

3. Encourage the child to breathe in and out slowly and gently. This will make a 'clicking' sound as the valve opens and closes.

4. Once the breathing pattern is well established, depress the canister with the free hand and leave the device in the same position as the child continues to breathe several more times. The child should take approximately 4-5 breaths for each puff of medication.

5. Remove the device from the child's mouth.

6. For a second dose wait a few seconds and repeat sections 1-5.

7. This device can also be used with the single breath technique in teenagers and adults.

Nebuhaler

**ALWAYS DEMONSTRATE TO THE PATIENT
HOW TO USE THE NEBUHALER**

© National Respiratory Traini

**Figure 4.16**
How to use the Nebuhaler.

**HOW TO USE THE NEBUCHAMBER**

1. Remove the protective cap from the aerosol inhaler.

2. Shake the inhaler so the contents are well mixed.

3. Place the mouthpiece of the aerosol inhaler into the small oval opening of the spacer.

4. Keeping the spacer level, place the mouthpiece between your teeth and close your lips around it.

5. Press (activate) the inhaler canister once and breathe in slowly and deeply through your mouth.

6. Hold your breath for about 10 seconds.

7. For each additonal dose of inhaler medication, remove the inhaler from the spacer and repeat steps 2-6.

8. Remove the inhaler from the spacer and replace the protective inhaler cap.

9. Replace spacer in storage bag.

NB. It may be preferable and easier for young children to take five breaths in and out (tidal breathing) to each actuation. The elderly may find it easier too.

**ALWAYS DEMONSTRATE TO THE PATIENT
HOW TO USE THE NEBUCHAMBER**

© National Respiratory Training Centre

Nebuchamber

**Figure 4.17**
How to use the Nebuchamber.

## HOW TO USE THE AEROCHAMBER

**Method for patient who can use the device without help**

1. Remove the cap.
2. Shake the inhaler and insert in the back of the Aerochamber.
3. Place the mouthpiece in the mouth.
4. Press the canister once to release a dose of the drug.
5. Take a deep, slow breath in. (If you hear a whistling sound, you are breathing in too quickly.)
6. Hold the breath for about ten seconds, then breathe out through the mouthpiece.
7. Breathe in again but do not press the canister.
8. Remove the mouthpiece from the mouth and breathe out.
9. Wait a few seconds before a second dose is taken, and repeat steps 2-8.

**Method particularly useful for young children**

1. Remove the cap.
2. Shake the inhaler and insert in the back of the Aerochamber.
3. Place the mouthpiece in the mouth.
4. Encourage the child to gently breathe in and out. (If you hear a whistling sound the child is breathing in too quickly*.)
5. Once the breathing pattern is well established, depress the canister with the free hand and leave the canister in the same position as the child continues to breathe in and out slowly five more times.
6. Remove the Aerochamber from the child's mouth.
7. For a second dose wait a few seconds and repeat steps 2-6.

   * NB. The child Aerochamber device with mask & infant Aerochamber device with mask do not whistle.

Aerochamber

**ALWAYS DEMONSTRATE TO THE PATIENT HOW TO USE AEROCHAMBER**

© National Respiratory Training C

**Figure 4.18**
How to use the Aerochamber.

## HOW TO USE A POCKET CHAMBER

1. Remove the mouthpiece cap from both the Pocket Chamber and the metered dose inhaler (MDI).
2. Place the MDI into the flexible end of the Pocket Chamber, which does not have the cap attached.
3. Make sure that you push it in fully.
4. Shake the spacer and MDI together 2 or 3 times.
5. Breathe out normally before placing the mouthpiece of the Pocket Chamber in your mouth. Close your lips tightly around the mouthpiece.
6. Depress the canister once, releasing one dose of medication. Breathe in slowly and fully. If you hear the 'coaching' whistle device on the spacer you are breathing in too hard.
7. Alternatively you can breathe in and out through the device about 5 times (multiple breath technique or tidal breathing). Remember the whistle should not be activated.
8. Remove the spacer from your mouth. If you have taken a single breath in, continue to hold your breath for about 5-10 seconds. Breathe out.
9. After use, remove the MDI from the spacer and replace the cap on the MDI as well as the cap on the Pocket Chamber.
10. Repeat steps 4-7 for further doses.

**ALWAYS DEMONSTRATE TO THE PATIENT HOW TO USE A POCKET CHAMBER**

Pocket Chamber

© National Respiratory Training Centre

**Figure 4.19**
How to use the Pocket Chamber.

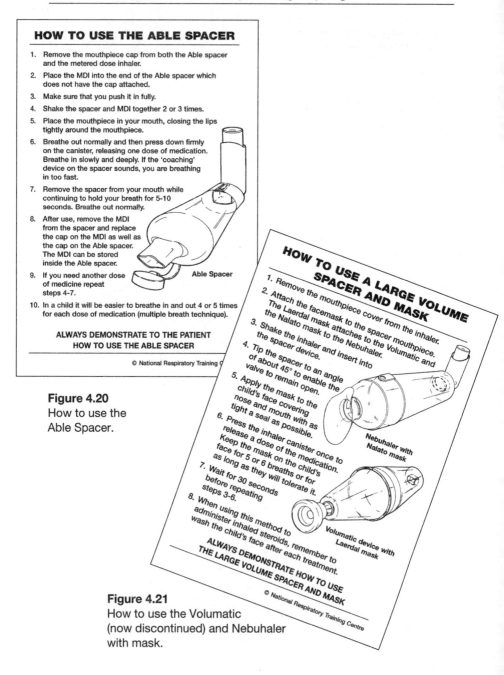

**HOW TO USE THE ABLE SPACER**

1. Remove the mouthpiece cap from both the Able spacer and the metered dose inhaler.

2. Place the MDI into the end of the Able spacer which does not have the cap attached.

3. Make sure that you push it in fully.

4. Shake the spacer and MDI together 2 or 3 times.

5. Place the mouthpiece in your mouth, closing the lips tightly around the mouthpiece.

6. Breathe out normally and then press down firmly on the canister, releasing one dose of medication. Breathe in slowly and deeply. If the 'coaching' device on the spacer sounds, you are breathing in too fast.

7. Remove the spacer from your mouth while continuing to hold your breath for 5-10 seconds. Breathe out normally.

8. After use, remove the MDI from the spacer and replace the cap on the MDI as well as the cap on the Able spacer. The MDI can be stored inside the Able spacer.

9. If you need another dose of medicine repeat steps 4-7.

Able Spacer

10. In a child it will be easier to breathe in and out 4 or 5 times for each dose of medication (multiple breath technique).

**ALWAYS DEMONSTRATE TO THE PATIENT HOW TO USE THE ABLE SPACER**

© National Respiratory Training C

**Figure 4.20**
How to use the Able Spacer.

**HOW TO USE A LARGE VOLUME SPACER AND MASK**

1. Remove the mouthpiece cover from the inhaler.

2. Attach the facemask to the spacer mouthpiece. The Laerdal mask attaches to the Volumatic and the Nalato mask to the Nebuhaler.

3. Shake the inhaler and insert into the spacer device.

4. Tip the spacer to an angle of about 45° to enable the valve to remain open.

5. Apply the mask to the child's face covering nose and mouth with as tight a seal as possible.

6. Press the inhaler canister once to release a dose of the medication. Keep the mask on the child's face for 5 or 6 breaths or for as long as they will tolerate it.

7. Wait for 30 seconds before repeating steps 3-6.

8. When using this method to administer inhaled steroids, remember to wash the child's face after each treatment.

Nebuhaler with Nalato mask

Volumatic device with Laerdal mask

**ALWAYS DEMONSTRATE HOW TO USE THE LARGE VOLUME SPACER AND MASK**

© National Respiratory Training Centre

**Figure 4.21**
How to use the Volumatic (now discontinued) and Nebuhaler with mask.

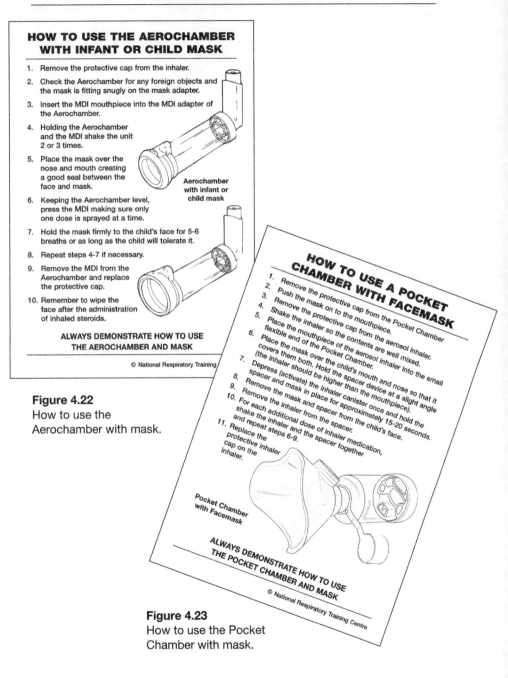

**HOW TO USE THE AEROCHAMBER WITH INFANT OR CHILD MASK**

1. Remove the protective cap from the inhaler.

2. Check the Aerochamber for any foreign objects and the mask is fitting snugly on the mask adapter.

3. Insert the MDI mouthpiece into the MDI adapter of the Aerochamber.

4. Holding the Aerochamber and the MDI shake the unit 2 or 3 times.

5. Place the mask over the nose and mouth creating a good seal between the face and mask.

6. Keeping the Aerochamber level, press the MDI making sure only one dose is sprayed at a time.

7. Hold the mask firmly to the child's face for 5-6 breaths or as long as the child will tolerate it.

8. Repeat steps 4-7 if necessary.

9. Remove the MDI from the Aerochamber and replace the protective cap.

10. Remember to wipe the face after the administration of inhaled steroids.

Aerochamber with infant or child mask

**ALWAYS DEMONSTRATE HOW TO USE THE AEROCHAMBER AND MASK**

© National Respiratory Training

**Figure 4.22**
How to use the
Aerochamber with mask.

**HOW TO USE A POCKET CHAMBER WITH FACEMASK**

1. Remove the protective cap from the Pocket Chamber

2. Push the mask on to the mouthpiece.

3. Remove the protective cap from the aerosol inhaler.

4. Shake the inhaler so the contents are well mixed.

5. Place the mouthpiece of the aerosol inhaler into the small flexible end of the Pocket Chamber.

6. Place the mask over the child's mouth and nose so that it covers them both. Hold the spacer device at a slight angle (the inhaler should be higher than the mouthpiece).

7. Depress (activate) the inhaler canister once and hold the spacer and mask in place for approximately 15-20 seconds.

8. Remove the mask and spacer from the child's face.

9. Remove the inhaler from the spacer.

10. For each additional dose of inhaler medication, shake the inhaler and the spacer together and repeat steps 6-9.

11. Replace the protective inhaler cap on the inhaler.

Pocket Chamber with Facemask

**ALWAYS DEMONSTRATE HOW TO USE THE POCKET CHAMBER AND MASK**

© National Respiratory Training Centre

**Figure 4.23**
How to use the Pocket
Chamber with mask.

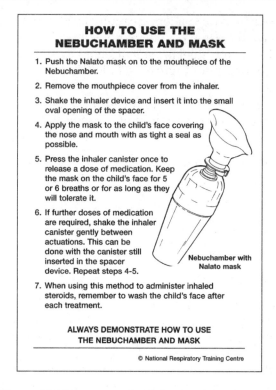

**HOW TO USE THE
NEBUCHAMBER AND MASK**

1. Push the Nalato mask on to the mouthpiece of the Nebuchamber.

2. Remove the mouthpiece cover from the inhaler.

3. Shake the inhaler device and insert it into the small oval opening of the spacer.

4. Apply the mask to the child's face covering the nose and mouth with as tight a seal as possible.

5. Press the inhaler canister once to release a dose of medication. Keep the mask on the child's face for 5 or 6 breaths or for as long as they will tolerate it.

6. If further doses of medication are required, shake the inhaler canister gently between actuations. This can be done with the canister still inserted in the spacer device. Repeat steps 4-5.

Nebuchamber with Nalato mask

7. When using this method to administer inhaled steroids, remember to wash the child's face after each treatment.

**ALWAYS DEMONSTRATE HOW TO USE
THE NEBUCHAMBER AND MASK**

© National Respiratory Training Centre

**Figure 4.24** How to use the Nebuchamber with mask.

## I'm being told different things about washing my spacer device. I'm not sure what to do.

Unfortunately there is still some confusion among health professionals about how to look after spacer devices. This means that people are told different things – which, as you say, is really confusing.

Plastic spacers attract a lot of static charge, which means that things 'stick' to the surface. In the case of inhaler medicines, when they are sprayed into the spacer, the medicine spray is attracted to the inside of the plastic spacer wall and sticks to it. This means that less medicine is available for you to breathe in through the spacer. All plastic type spacers currently available on prescription in the UK have the same problem with static charge. Spacers that are made of stainless steel are not affected by static charge. In the UK the Nebuchamber (Figure 4.17) is the only device made of stainless steel.

Research has looked at the different ways we wash spacer devices. The result has shown that we should wash them in the following way:

1. Separate the two halves of large spacers or take off the removable coloured ends of the small spacers.

2. Wash in warm soapy water (washing-up liquid is fine).

3. Leave to soak for a few minutes.

4. Drip dry without rinsing.

5. Reassemble when dry.

The detergent that dries on the spacer acts as an antistatic coating and stops the inhaler medicine sticking to the plastic. **Do not rinse and do not dry the spacer with a tissue or cloth as this will increase the static charge.**

You need to wash your spacer device only every 3–4 weeks because the antistatic effects of the detergent coating last for this amount of time.

## Side effects

We have received many questions about side effects of asthma medicines. We have tried to answer your questions as honestly as we can. No medicine is entirely free of side effects, and we feel that we are probably more likely to have had questions from those people unlucky enough to get them, rather than the majority who do not. Our message is that most anti-asthma medicines used today are safe and largely free from side effects. Troublesome side effects are confined to a very few people, usually those who require higher dosages, because of the severity of their condition.

### Is it safe to use more than the stated dose of my blue inhaler?

It won't hurt you in the short term, but the important thing is to know why you need to take more than the stated dose. Your blue inhaler is a reliever, works within a few minutes and is usually very effective. It contains medicines that relax the tightness in muscles in your airways. Your blue inhaler contains either salbutamol (e.g. Ventolin) or terbutaline (Bricanyl). If your asthma is becoming more severe, you will find that it becomes less effective. It may be tempting to keep on taking puffs of your Ventolin or Bricanyl (even though it doesn't seem to be doing much good) but this can be dangerous. If it is losing its effect, you should seek medical help, either from your GP or asthma nurse or from the hospital. Once your airways have become very inflamed and narrow, Ventolin or Bricanyl has very little effect. Other medicines such as steroid tablets are then needed to treat your asthma and you may need to take a regular steroid inhaler medicine as well as other treatments.

The aim of asthma treatment is to prevent symptoms from occurring, in turn reducing the need to take extra blue inhaler medicine.

### How can long-term complications of treatments be balanced against the short-term benefits that they give?

It is always difficult to balance what gives pleasure today against the problems that may occur in the future (a good example of this is cigarette smoking). Your question suggests that this balance needs to be made in asthma, and we agree. You may have to balance the 'pleasure' of no symptoms today, by taking treatment, against possible long-term side effects of that treatment. On the other hand you may feel that you prefer to take no treatment, and run the risk of dangerous asthma attacks at any time, and long-term damage to your lungs later in life. This can be a difficult decision to take, and you need help from your asthma nurse or doctor to let you decide what the right course is.

There is no doubt that asthma causes troublesome symptoms and many studies have confirmed this. However, many people do not realize the extent to which asthma is interfering with their lives. Approximately half of the 61 000 people responding to a national survey reported that they had symptoms from asthma every day of their lives. Most of these simply accepted that such symptoms are part of life, and they put up with the problems caused by them. This need not be the case with present-day treatments. The benefits of asthma treatment, such as improving the quality of life, are immense.

We consider that the evidence is strongly in favour of the long-term safety of the medicines we use today, in inhaled form and in standard dosages. That is why we believe the advantages of short- and long-term treatment considerably outweigh any possible long-term complications of treatment. This is such an important issue for all asthmatics that we urge you to discuss it with all those involved in your asthma care.

## What are the side effects of inhaled relievers?

All of the side effects with relievers are temporary, and occur only while the medicine is being taken. If you are taking relievers by inhaler and in normal doses, then very few side effects are likely. Any that you notice will be only temporary. Relievers such as salbutamol (Ventolin), terbutaline (Bricanyl), and the longer acting medicines salmeterol (Serevent) and formoterol (Foradil and Oxis) can cause a fine trembling (tremor) of the muscles, particularly in the hands. This side effect usually wears off within a few minutes, or hours at most. If higher doses of these medicines are used, the pulse rate may increase, and palpitations (or pounding) of the heart may be noticed. This is not harmful but may be an unpleasant sensation.

Another group of relievers, called anticholinergic medicines, work in a different way, and tend to have different side effects. The best known of this group is ipratropium bromide (Atrovent), but they are now recommended only for the treatment of acute severe asthma. Again, the side effects are very few but will increase with higher doses, particularly in nebulizer form. People may notice that their mouth becomes dry, and their vision blurred. Rarely, it may be difficult to pass urine, and constipation may occur.

**Ventolin appears to work instantly for me, but what tissue damage is occurring?**

None. On its own Ventolin is simply a reliever medicine and certainly doesn't cause any damage. It helps to open up tightened airways and should work instantly, or at least within a few minutes, and this relief should normally last at least 4 hours. It is a suitable treatment for people with very mild asthma who need only occasional relief medication. The current advice is that, preferably, Ventolin should not be used regularly. This inhaler medicine (as well as Bricanyl and other inhaled relievers) should normally be used only when you have respiratory symptoms.

If you need to use Ventolin or Bricanyl every day, it is a warning sign that you need to start preventer treatment or you need additional preventer treatment to keep your asthma under better control. **If your reliever medicine does not work quickly, or its effects last for less than 4 hours, your asthma is uncontrolled and medical help is needed. Take extra reliever while waiting for help or advice.** This very important point is dealt with in Chapter 8 on *Emergencies*.

**Are any of these inhalers addictive?**

No. Many people, particularly parents of children with asthma, worry that inhalers may be addictive. They fear that the more treatment you take, the more you will need. As a result they allow themselves, or their children, to suffer unpleasant symptoms that could have been avoided if the asthma treatment had been given. This concern is misplaced. Asthma medicines are not addictive and you do not need to keep increasing the dose to get the same effect. If anything the reverse is true, and asthma left untreated now may lead to larger amounts of medicines being required in the future, as well as to a permanent narrowing of the airways.

We all want to see maximum effect from the minimum treatment needed, but sometimes it is necessary to take higher doses to get good control over the asthma. This is not because treatment is addictive, but because the asthma has become worse.

**I don't want to become dependent on my inhalers. Will this happen if I take them regularly?**

You won't become dependent on your asthma inhalers. The reliever inhalers (e.g. Ventolin and Bricanyl) are generally best taken on an 'as required' basis rather than regularly. If they are taken regularly (and by this we mean perhaps 4–6 times a day), you may become more reliant on them. This is not because the medicine is addictive, but because they are probably being relied upon to give you relief from your asthma symptoms. Nowadays it is thought best to take preventer treatment if a reliever medicine is needed more than once a day.

To keep your asthma well controlled your asthma doctor or nurse may ask you to take some regular asthma preventer medicine. The preventer medicines (e.g. AeroBec, Alvesco, Asmabec, Asmanex, Becotide, Flixotide, Pulmicort, Pulvinal [beclometasone], Qvar) do not give immediate relief and you need only to take them either once or twice a day. Preventer medicines will control the inflammation within the airways but you will not become dependent on them.

**Aren't steroids harmful?**

The steroids used to treat asthma are generally very safe. We should first make it clear that the steroids used in asthma treatment are not the same as the steroids abused by a few athletes. Those are called *anabolic* (or sex hormone) *steroids*. In asthma we are concerned with a type called corticosteroids.

Corticosteroids have a major role in the treatment of asthma. They are given in different ways – by the inhaled route, by mouth (oral) or occasionally by injection. Very low doses are needed if they are given by the inhaled route, and in standard doses almost none of the medicine is absorbed into the body. Side effects in these circumstances are uncommon.

Steroid injections are not often needed these days. They are nearly always reserved for acute attacks of asthma, particularly if someone is vomiting and unable to swallow tablets. On the other hand, steroid tablets are frequently given to control acute asthma attacks. A short course of tablets, even in high doses, will have few side effects. Occasionally people notice some weight gain, or a mood change, but the effects are temporary. The advantages in taking a short course of steroids for an acute attack far outweigh the disadvantages. They can be life saving.

In people with severe asthma, taking steroid tablets long term, that is over months or years, can have serious side effects. These side effects include weight gain, particularly a fullness of the face ('moon face'), and a thinning of the skin, which leads to easy bruising. The blood pressure may increase, and there is a greater risk of developing diabetes in those prone to it. Other problems may be stomach ulcers and thinning of the bones. These problems are not common, but all are recognized long-term risks with oral steroids. This is why, wherever possible, inhaled rather than oral steroids medicines are given. There is some concern that very high doses of the inhaled steroids may cause some of these same effects over many years, but the evidence for normal dosages is very reassuring. It emphasizes how important it is always to use as low a dose of corticosteroids as possible.

**Are there any side effects from inhaled steroids?**

When taken in low doses the only serious side effect of *topical (inhaled) steroids* is hoarseness of the voice but very few people are affected. It reverses if the treatment is stopped. The other problem can be thrush of the mouth (otherwise known as candida infection), which may cause soreness and an unpleasant taste in the mouth. Both problems can be prevented by using your inhaler before brushing your teeth, and by rinsing your mouth out very well.

Both problems are more likely to occur at higher doses of inhaled steroid medicines. With thrush, the back of the throat becomes sore and is red with white spots. This can irritate or cause voice problems. You can usually avoid this by using a spacer device (Volumatic [now discontinued – Figures 4.14 and 4.15], Nebuhaler [Figure 4.16]. Nebuchamber [Figure 4.17], Aerochamber [Figure 4.18], Pocket Chamber [Figure 4.19] or Able Spacer [Figure 4.20]) with your pressurized inhaler. The spacer device acts as a holding chamber for the dose of medicine, which is released when the inhaler canister is pressed. The spacer prevents the medicine spray hitting the back of the throat. Sometimes eating live natural yoghurt (which acts against the thrush) every day may help.

The newer steroid medicine called ciclesonide (Alvesco), is inactive in the mouth and only works once it reaches the lungs. This medicine may be useful where persistent oral thrush occurs. If very high doses of steroid inhalers are used over many years, there may be a small risk of thinning of the bones (*osteoporosis*). However, very high doses are required only when the alternatives are to have dangerously uncontrolled asthma, or to take steroid tablets long term.

### Will the steroids stunt my child's growth?

Steroid medicines do not stunt the growth if they are used at normal doses. Rather than use the term 'stunting', it is better to talk about delaying growth. Occasional short courses of oral steroids, such as prednisolone, will not affect your child's growth even when they are given in high doses. They are essential in the management of an acute asthma attack, and can be life saving. If these short courses are required several times each year, or if steroid tablets have to be taken over a long period of time, e.g. months or years, they can have some effect on growth, but so does poorly controlled asthma.

The introduction of inhaled steroids in the early 1970s made a tremendous difference and meant that asthma could be well controlled, without the risks of long-term oral steroids. Despite this, there has still been concern that inhaled steroids might have an unfavourable effect on growth, if given to children over a number of years. Research has been carried out on the effects of long-term inhaled steroids medicines and children's growth. Contrary to many worries, growth actually improved in many children, because the asthma was better controlled.

If higher doses of inhaled steroids (800 μg beclometasone or more per day) are used, side effects are more likely. A balance must be drawn between the known effect of uncontrolled asthma in reducing children's growth, and the possible effect of high-dose inhaled steroids in doing the same. If high doses of inhaled steroid are needed, your child should be under the care of a children's doctor who specializes in asthma.

**I am 72 years old and have been told that my osteoporosis has probably got worse because I have been on Ventolin and Becotide for many years. Is this true?**

Osteoporosis is a gradual thinning and weakening of the bones owing to a loss of calcium from the body. It occurs in all people to some extent as they become older. It results in an increased tendency to fractures, particularly of the hips and spine. Sometimes it is made worse as a side effect of steroid tablets but usually only after years of use. It is unlikely that your osteoporosis has become worse owing to your Becotide, unless you have been taking very high doses for several years or more. If you have, it is also likely that you may have needed many short courses of steroid tablets for acute asthma, and the cumulative effect of these may have contributed to your osteoporosis. Ventolin does not have any effect whatsoever on osteoporosis.

It is worth bearing in mind that all women who have passed the menopause may develop osteoporosis anyway. It occurs more often in smokers and those who do not take exercise. Hormone replacement therapy given during and after the menopause will help to retain the body's calcium stores and may prevent osteoporosis, but that treatment itself has to be balanced against the risk of other long-term side effects. There are also some very effective bone protection medicines that can be used. A family history of osteoporosis is in itself a risk factor for developing osteoporosis.

**Why can't I take prednisolone all the time?**

We have some sympathy with your question. Taking prednisolone (steroid) tablets on a regular basis to keep your asthma well controlled all the time seems, on the face of it, to be a very attractive suggestion. Some people see it as a way of not having to use regular preventer inhalers. So why don't we recommend long-term use of prednisolone, unless it is absolutely essential? The reason is because of important side effects.

Taking prednisolone continuously means that the level of steroid in the blood is always high. Because of this the *adrenal glands* make less *cortisol*, which is the body's natural equivalent of prednisolone. Eventually after long-term (not short-term) use the adrenal gland becomes inactive. It stops producing cortisol itself, and the body comes to rely completely on the steroid tablets. Cortisol is produced by the body to cope with all kinds of stress, for example a serious illness. If the steroid tablets are stopped suddenly for some reason, the adrenal glands cannot make up the difference. In this case, the body is dangerously prone to illness. This is why people taking long-term steroid tablet treatment need to carry warning cards to show to any doctor who might be treating them.

There are other serious side effects that can occur if prednisolone is taken over many years. These include skin changes, thinning of the bones, increases in blood pressure, indigestion and ulcers, and the development of diabetes. This is an alarming list, and we must emphasize that these risks are not present with the use of short courses of prednisolone, which are important for treating uncontrolled and acute asthma, unless a large number of such courses are required over a number of years.

A small number of people with chronic severe asthma do find that inhaled steroids, even in high doses, are not sufficient to control symptoms. In these cases doctors have little choice but to prescribe regular doses of steroid tablets. Side effects are much more likely to occur in these cases if the dose needed is above 5 mg/day, taken over a long period of time. Those with severe asthma need to be under the care of a specialist chest doctor so their asthma can be carefully monitored.

### Why do I keep getting white spots on the back of my throat?

It is likely that you have thrush infection in your throat. This is also known as *candida* or *monilia infection*, but is best known as thrush. It is a fungus infection, and is one of the very few side effects caused by inhaled steroids. Fortunately thrush can be treated effectively using an antifungal treatment in liquid or lozenge form.

The chances of it recurring can be reduced in several ways. The simplest is to rinse out your mouth and clean your teeth whenever you use your preventer inhaler. Another way, particularly when higher doses are prescribed, is to use a spacer device (e.g. Volumatic [now discontinued – Figures 4.14 and 4.15], Nebuhaler [Figure 4.16], Nebuchamber [Figure 4.17], Aerochamber [Figure 4.18], Pocket Chamber [Figure 4.19] or Able Spacer [Figure 4.20]). These devices allow the larger particles of the medicines (which are the likely cause of thrush) to be held in the holding chamber, rather than be deposited in the mouth and throat. Spacers also prevent the spray hitting the back of the throat. We have already mentioned a newer steroid medicine ciclesonide (Alvesco), which is inactive in the mouth and therefore may reduce the side effects of thrush. Perhaps talk to your doctor or asthma nurse about this.

### Does any of my asthma medication affect my immune system?

This depends on your treatment(s) and the dosage. Very few people with asthma have to take so much treatment that their immune system is affected, but it is possible. Steroid tablets (prednisolone) taken over a long period of time can affect the immune system. The result of this is that someone may suffer more infections than normal, or may not be able to fight infections as effectively as other people. One way of reducing the risk of prednisolone side effects is to take the tablets on alternate days rather than every day. There are no effects on the immune system if you need to take only occasional short courses of steroid tablets each year.

In theory at least, inhaled steroids in very high doses may also pose a risk to the immune system, although there is little or no evidence to confirm this. High doses in adults are generally agreed to be above 800 µg/day of Becotide (beclometasone) or Pulmicort (budesonide), and above 400 µg/day of Asmanex (mometasone) or Flixotide (fluticasone). In children half of the above daily doses are considered to be high and a children's chest specialist opinion is probably advisable for children taking these doses. Fortunately not many people need such high doses. It is better to use a spacer device for delivering high doses of inhaled steroids because it reduces the local side effects and ensures effective delivery of the medicine to the lungs.

**I read in the paper that asthma treatments are dangerous. Is this true?**

Asthma treatments are not dangerous but asthma itself can be if it is not controlled. In low doses there are no serious side effects from any of the asthma medicines. As the doses are increased, then the risks of side effects are greater. However, doses are only increased when asthma is not controlled or is getting worse, and therefore people are at more risk from the condition itself.

High doses of steroids over long periods of time may cause side effects, whether taken in tablet form or by the inhaled route. The most serious of these are a reduced ability to fight infections and thinning of the bones (osteoporosis). If you are taking high doses of inhaled steroid medicines, these risks can be reduced by using a spacer device such as a Volumatic [now discontinued – Figures 4.14 and 4.15], Nebuhaler [Figure 4.16], Nebuchamber [Figure 4.17], Aerochamber [Figure 4.18], Pocket Chamber [Figure 4.19] or Able Spacer [Figure 4.20].

Theophylline medicines (*aminophylline*, Nuelin, Slo-Phyllin, Uniphyllin) are used less often now as other medicines are more effective, but they may be dangerous if the levels in the blood are too high. Anyone taking these medicines should have a blood test from time to time to check that the levels are satisfactory. Some medicines such as cimetidine (Tagamet) or erythromycin (an antibiotic) increase the risk of problems with theophyllines. Always check with your doctor or asthma nurse if you are prescribed these medicines.

Make sure that you have a regular asthma review with your doctor or asthma nurse. This may need to be only once or twice a year if all is going well. However, if your symptoms are worsening, you might need additional asthma medicines or to increase your existing treatments. Generally the aim is for you to control your asthma with the lowest possible dose of a medicine. This is covered in Chapter 5 ***Beating asthma***.

**I have a young child who has asthma. What does Ventolin syrup do?**

Ventolin syrup is a reliever medicine, which is swallowed rather than inhaled. The active medicine is exactly the same as Ventolin (generic name salbutamol) that is taken in inhalers or nebulizers. However, it needs to be taken in a higher dose than by the inhaled route, because it has to be taken into the bloodstream from the stomach and circulated all round the body before reaching the lungs. Inhaled Ventolin goes straight to the lungs and not into the bloodstream which is why it is the preferred choice. The side effects of Ventolin syrup are shaking (or trembling) of the hands, and pounding (or racing) of the heart. These are the same side effects that some people feel when they take a lot of Ventolin through their inhaler. A few children may become hyperactive when taking Ventolin syrup. Side effects always disappear if the medicine is stopped.

**Will steroids affect my teenage daughter's growth?**

They could do, but it depends on how she takes them, what dose she takes and for how long. It's important to look at the different aspects of treating asthma with steroids, and to take them one by one.

First, if steroid tablets are given to children for **a long time** (**months or longer**) they do slow down growth temporarily. There are very few children who require steroid tablets to this extent. In those who do, growth is less likely to be affected if the steroid tablets are taken on alternate days.

Second, low-dose inhaled steroids are extremely effective as preventive agents. At usual doses it is known that they will not have any effect on a child's growth. Care must be taken when higher doses are needed to control the asthma. When inhaled steroid dosages are increased on a long-term basis, it is important to weigh up all considerations. We should always aim to give minimal treatment for maximum effect. If the higher doses of inhaled steroids are needed, then the use of spacer devices will reduce the risk of side effects, including the slowing down of growth. It is important to monitor every child's growth during the course of their asthma treatment, especially if they are on any steroid medicines.

Third, remember that uncontrolled chronic asthma itself does cause a slowing down of growth. In fact, the introduction of inhaled steroids often means that growth increases because asthma symptoms improve.

Finally, it is interesting that many children with asthma have a delayed puberty, and their adolescent growth spurt is held up. Once puberty and the growth spurt do occur, the eventual height reached is at least that predicted from their earlier growth performance, and can be above average.

### Does my blue inhaler affect tooth enamel?

A blue inhaler contains your reliever medicine and is unlikely to affect your teeth. Although most of the dry powder inhalers contain lactose, which is a type of sugar, the amount is so small that it is unlikely to cause tooth decay. Tooth enamel is damaged by sugar because the sugar ferments in your mouth and produces acid, and the acid then attacks the enamel. Lactose tends to be less harmful than the sugars we put into tea or coffee, or which we eat in sweets and biscuits. You can reduce any risk to your teeth by cleaning them after using your inhaler. Try to fit this into your night and morning routine.

### Can inhaled steroids make children hyperactive and cause sleep problems?

Not that we are aware of, but in medicine even the most unlikely things can happen! Steroid tablets taken in high doses can occasionally cause side effects such as mood changes, nightmares and mental disturbances. However, it is very rare indeed for inhaled steroids to have any sort of effect on the central nervous system. A few cases of unusual mood changes in patients taking beclometasone (Becotide or Becloforte) have been reported, but it does not necessarily mean that they were caused by the medicine. The events may have occurred for other reasons in those people.

The incidence of serious side effects for people using inhaled steroids is very low. This risk must be compared with the positive benefits obtained from their use.

### Why is my asthma control poor?

It is difficult to answer this question without more detail, because there are several common reasons for asthma to become uncontrolled. These reasons include:

- not being able to use your inhaler device correctly
- not taking your inhaler regularly
- not having the right asthma treatment
- needing some more asthma treatment
- being exposed to a new asthma trigger that is making your asthma worse.

Sometimes it is easy to sort out, such as making sure you can use your inhaler correctly. This may mean that your inhaler device is changed to something you can use. There may be other reasons why your asthma control is poor. Your asthma nurse or doctor may ask you to do your peak flow blowing tests on a day-to-day basis for a few weeks to help them have a better understanding of your asthma control. It is possible that your asthma medicines need to be changed, either in dosage or perhaps some additional medicines prescribed. You may even need a short course of oral steroids to gain rapid control of your asthma.

**I am really worried about my son who has just been diagnosed with asthma. The specialist at the hospital wants to put him on Flixotide but the leaflet inside the packet says it's for children over the age of 4. He's only 2.**

We understand your concerns about your son, especially if you have just found out that he has asthma. The good thing is that he is being seen by a specialist at the hospital who will have made sure that there is nothing else wrong with your son. Flixotide (fluticasone) is an inhaled steroid medicine which will help to control your son's asthma. Asthma medicines such as Flixotide are sometimes used 'off-label' in younger children. This means that when the medicine was licensed by the medicine safety authorities, research studies had not been carried out in younger children. The product licence for this medicine could therefore only state that it was for use in children from 4 years of age; it does not mean that the medicine is unsafe. Carrying out research in children and pregnant women is always difficult because there are ethical and practical issues to be considered.

We are sure that your doctor will have thought very carefully about the asthma medicines needed to improve your son's asthma. The doctor will also be aware of the recommended licensing age for Flixotide. The important thing is that your son is on preventer asthma treatment, which gives the best conditions to control his symptoms.

## New on the market

**I have read on the internet that there is a new injection treatment for asthma. Is this correct, as my local pharmacist was unsure just when it was going to be available in the UK?**

You are right, there is a new injection treatment but it was originally available only in the USA. It is used to treat allergic asthma but only for those with more severe asthma. It is not a substitute for usual asthma treatments, but its use may allow lower doses to be used. It is an anti-immunoglobulin E (IgE) treatment and has just been licensed for use in the UK.

IgE is an antibody which is produced as part of the body's normal protective response to fight foreign inhaled proteins, such as pollen grains. In allergy-triggered asthma, IgE production is part of the allergic inflammatory process, which causes respiratory symptoms. This injection treatment blocks IgE and prevents the inflammation developing and the symptoms of asthma occurring.

It is an exciting treatment but it will be used initially only for adults and children over 12 years of age with more severe asthma. Injection treatment is given every 2 or 4 weeks, the dose depending on blood IgE levels and body weight. The new injection treatment is called omalizumab (Xolair). It is likely that initially it will only be prescribed by respiratory specialist doctors.

---

### Personal action plan – things you might wish to discuss with your doctor or asthma nurse

It is important to make sure that you are on the right medication to control your asthma. It is possible that your asthma is perfectly controlled but, if not, you may need a higher or lower dose, or you may need a different kind of inhaler device.

At your next asthma review, ask whether your medication needs to be changed or altered. The following information would help in answering your question. When your asthma is worse tell the doctor or asthma nurse:

- what sort of symptoms you are having, particularly at night or on exercise
- what inhaler medicines you are taking and how often
- how much your asthma is troubling you
- what your peak flow readings (blowing tests) are like, and
- what your peak flow chart is like.

It is very helpful if you do a peak flow chart for the week before you go for your check-up, and take the chart with you.

# 5

# Beating asthma

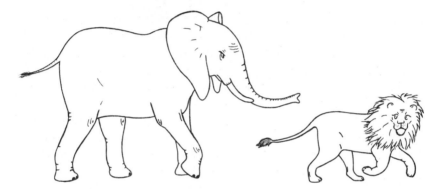

---

**In this chapter you will learn about:**

- why asthma doesn't have to control your life

- how asthma can be controlled

- how to keep a check on your asthma (monitoring control)

- when to monitor your asthma

- what the warning signs are when asthma is out of control

- how you can help yourself

- when to call for help.

---

Success in looking after your asthma depends on knowing what makes up good (and poor) asthma control. This allows you to make changes to your treatment in response to changes in your asthma symptoms. Getting the treatment right in the first place is a result of the partnership between you and your doctor, your asthma nurse and other health professionals, who may be involved in helping you to manage your asthma. Once you have been prescribed treatment, you are the person who has to live with your asthma and recognize when symptoms change.

We believe that the best ways to monitor asthma are to use symptoms **and** peak expiratory flow readings (if you are able to use a peak flow meter). Peak flow readings are sometimes referred to as a 'blowing test' but in this chapter we will use the term peak flow readings. Peak flow meters are available on National Health Service prescriptions in the UK. All peak flow meters give slightly different results; therefore it is best to have your own. If you can, take it with you when you go for an asthma check with your asthma nurse or doctor.

There are many people with peak flow meters who take their readings only occasionally because for them it is inconvenient to measure it every day. Although this is better than not recording it all, regular measurement will provide valuable information because peak flow readings often change before there are obvious symptoms of uncontrolled asthma. If you cannot or don't want to do your peak flow readings every day, record them when you have a cold or when you have asthma symptoms. These readings will help you decide what extra asthma treatment you need and when to seek help. Your asthma nurse and doctor can work out with you when your peak flow readings are OK and when they are not. This information can be written down on an asthma action plan for you to look at when you need to check what to do.

In the UK in 2002 there were 69 000 hospital admissions for acute asthma. Many of these asthma attacks and hospital admissions could be avoided by quick action and the right treatment, provided that the attack is recognized early. We believe that helping you to recognize *uncontrolled asthma* is one of the most important functions of this book. Uncontrolled asthma means danger and we urge you to read this section carefully.

One of the biggest changes in asthma care in recent years has been the introduction of asthma action plans for all people with asthma. Asthma action plans are sometimes known as self-management plans. Action plans can vary from being a list of your asthma medicines and when to take them, to more complicated action plans, using peak flow readings or starting a course of steroid tablets for acute asthma. We know that asthma action plans can help you look after your asthma and all people with asthma should have one. Your asthma nurse or doctor can help you to develop your own action plan.

## What is my responsibility in looking after me and my asthma?

We all have some responsibilities to ourselves and our health. If you have asthma, learning about asthma is very helpful. You need to learn how it is treated and when to call for help. While many children apparently 'grow out of their asthma', it is a condition that stays for life. There may be times, sometimes lasting several years, when it doesn't cause any problems and we say that the asthma has gone into remission. Unfortunately, symptoms can return or flare up and it is helpful to be able to recognize this. As with many other situations in life, knowing what to do to make things better will help you be in control.

The main things you can do are to:

- avoid triggers that make your asthma worse

- see your doctor or asthma nurse for regular check-ups

- take your medication as advised

- learn how to recognize when your asthma is going out of control and what to do if that happens.

Many of these things are discussed in this chapter; the rest can be found in other sections of this book.

## What can I do myself?

Probably the most important thing you can do is to keep yourself fit and well: 20–30 minutes of brisk walking every day, or other forms of exercise, will help to keep you fit. Eating sensibly and having a good healthy balanced diet is also essential; this should include some fruit and fresh vegetables every day. If you smoke, stopping smoking will be of enormous benefit to you both now and in the future. Smoke irritates the airways, stops your asthma medicines working well, increases respiratory illnesses in young children, causes lung cancer and is generally antisocial. It is also expensive!

It may seem very obvious to say this but, if you have been prescribed medicines for your asthma, it is best to take them. We frequently meet patients who have had an asthma attack because they have stopped taking or run out of their asthma medicines. This is as frustrating for us as professionals as for the sufferers, because we know that good asthma control can be achieved when asthma medicines are taken regularly. Asthma is a lifelong condition and most doctors and asthma nurses will set up a system to help you obtain repeat prescriptions of your asthma medicines, as well as an emergency supply of prednisolone tablets in case of asthma attacks. Your responsibility (or your carer's responsibility) is to make sure that the repeat prescription is ordered **before** the medicines run out. Repeat prescription systems vary from practice to practice, but they do have a few things in common. There are usually a set number of repeat prescriptions (repeats) that have been authorized by the practice before you need to see the doctor or asthma nurse for a check-up. This is usually set for 3–12 repeats, depending on how often you have asthma symptoms and how severe your asthma is.

Regular check-ups either at the surgery or in a dedicated asthma clinic give you the opportunity to discuss your asthma and to learn how you can recognize when your asthma is out of control. You can also learn how to deal with these episodes.

# Seeing the doctor, the asthma nurse – and asthma clinics

**Do I need to see my GP every time I think asthma is coming, or just use my inhaler?**

The answer to this question depends on a number of factors, of which two are perhaps the most important. These are:

- the severity of your asthma

- the type of inhaled asthma treatment you use.

Ideally, you should agree an asthma action plan (self-management plan) with your doctor or asthma nurse. This plan will deal with what should happen when your asthma symptoms get worse. Usually there will be one or more steps that you can take before, or in addition to, seeking help. It may be a simple step, such as increasing the dose of reliever inhaler. On the other hand it may be a number of steps, which may include starting a course of steroid tablets before you see your doctor or asthma nurse.

If you have an asthma attack, your asthma action plan and treatment should be reviewed with your doctor or asthma nurse, either in the general surgery or at an asthma clinic. It may be necessary to make some changes to your treatment to prevent another attack.

There is a section on action plans (self-management plans) later in this chapter.

**How often should I see my doctor or go to the clinic?**

This varies greatly, depending on the type and severity of your asthma. Some people suffer from asthma only during certain times of the year, for example in the hay fever season. In these cases, your asthma may need to be reviewed only once a year. On the other hand, people who have very severe asthma may need to attend the surgery or clinic every month or so.

There are some special times when it is particularly important to see the doctor or asthma nurse for review of your asthma. These are as follows:

- Everyone should be reviewed soon after an attack of asthma if it is severe enough to need a high dose of emergency bronchodilator or reliever medication. Regardless of whether such treatment took place in the surgery, at home or in hospital, an appointment should be booked as soon as possible. It is always difficult to predict how long an attack will take to clear up completely, but a daily peak flow chart will help you monitor your asthma. The review is an ideal time to discuss this chart and decide how to continue the treatment. Those involved can also try to work out why the attack occurred and decide what needs to be done in order to prevent another.

- An asthma check-up appointment before going on holiday is often helpful. Action plans are sometimes needed when you are on holiday and may even save lives. Spare inhaler prescriptions are a good idea if you are going away, especially if you are going abroad (see the section on *Written action plans for asthma* later).

**My doctor says I would benefit from attending his asthma clinic. What is this and what happens there?**

GPs frequently provide a range of clinics where particular conditions (such as asthma or diabetes) or particular problems (such as stopping smoking or preventing heart disease) are dealt with in one clinic rather than in the usual general surgeries. Some of these clinics are run by the GP, while others are run by the practice asthma nurse. In some cases both the GP and the asthma nurse run the clinic together. The main advantage of such clinics for asthma is that they usually provide more time to talk. There are many things to learn about asthma and these can't be dealt with easily in a busy surgery with 5- or 10-minute appointment times. The clinic setting allows more time to deal with questions or concerns, particularly for those people whose asthma has recently been diagnosed. This book is an attempt to answer many of the questions which crop up repeatedly, but it is also helpful to talk to someone who is experienced in dealing with asthma.

A major problem in asthma care comes from the difficulties in arranging regular follow-up and monitoring of people with asthma. These may occur because:

- the GP doesn't seem to have the time

- the GP doesn't think follow-up is needed

- the GP doesn't offer follow-up appointments

- the person with asthma doesn't take up the offer of an appointment

- the person with asthma feels well and fails to keep the appointment.

A GP's asthma clinic offers some solutions to these problems. It is often more convenient and less crowded than a hospital clinic. Community pharmacists are also beginning to be involved in sharing asthma care with the doctor and asthma nurse in some areas, which is an exciting development. The practice asthma nurse can check that the people on the practice *asthma register* are offered regular appointments to be seen, arrange 'flu vaccinations once a year, and make contact with people who do not attend.

**If you are on a practice's asthma register, how many people (such as future employers) have access to this information?**

All information about you on a computer is protected under the Data Protection Act. Nobody has access to this information without your permission. An asthma register is a document or computer file held by a practice in order to help organize its asthma care. It is confidential to the practice.

Your own medical record, which is held by your GP practice, is also strictly confidential. Information about your health cannot be given to anyone – by your GP or any of the practice staff – without your consent. In addition, you have the right to see that information before it is forwarded, with your permission, to an employer, an insurance company or anybody else, as long as you arrange to do so within 21 days of the request. If you are unwilling for the contents to be forwarded, you can ask for them to be withheld, although your GP will have to disclose that you have made this request.

Always ask to discuss this issue with your GP if you are concerned about other people having access to your medical details. Confidentiality is one of the most important parts of the relationship between health professionals and patients.

## Why do I need to come to a clinic?

There are many important aspects to asthma and its treatment. An asthma clinic in general practice should offer more time than the usual surgery appointments, and should be run by someone with a special interest and training in asthma. This extra time and experience offers obvious benefits to you and your family. Many hospitals also run asthma clinics now in preference to general chest clinics, and these have specially trained staff who can assist people with asthma in their understanding and management of the condition. These clinics may be asthma nurse-run or the more usual doctor and asthma nurse clinics.

Of course clinics vary from practice to practice and between hospitals. Generally though, they will concentrate on the following:

- answering questions and discussing concerns people may have about asthma
- helping people understand more about their asthma and the medicines used
- checking to make sure that the inhaler medicine is helpful
- making sure that the inhaler device that has been prescribed is suitable, in other words checking that you can use the device correctly
- teaching about the use of peak expiratory flow readings and charts

- helping people to prevent attacks because they have a better understanding of their asthma treatments and why peak flow meters are used

- helping people recognize when their asthma is going out of control, and how to deal with emergencies.

An asthma clinic should offer you the best possible opportunity for discussing your asthma and any concerns that you may have about your treatment or progress.

Some practices offer telephone follow-up appointments for people with asthma. These may be helpful if you cannot get to the surgery because of work commitments and if you only need advice. If your surgery does offer this service, make sure you get a prescription for a peak flow meter, find out how to use it, and keep a chart for a week before the telephone 'check-up'.

**I have had repeat prescriptions for several years now, and haven't seen my doctor. What shall I do?**

We advise you very strongly to see your doctor or asthma nurse. If your practice runs an asthma clinic, then ask to attend. If not, see them in surgery time. If your GP practice does not seem interested in asthma, and you are worried by your symptoms, ask to be referred to a specialist at your local hospital. Asthma treatments and the recommendations as to how asthma is treated do change as we learn more about it. Your treatment should be reviewed and may need to be changed in line with current treatment recommendations. Inhalers are not easy to use correctly so it is worth having your technique checked whenever you attend for an asthma review, in case you would be better switching to a different inhaler device.

Even if your asthma is mild, or you manage it very effectively by yourself, it is always good for the doctor and asthma nurse to see someone who is controlling their asthma successfully! It will also give you the satisfaction that you are doing things right and may even result in a reduction in the amount of asthma medicines you take.

### Can my husband be referred for tests to see what's causing his asthma?

Your question makes me think you would also like to know more about his asthma. If your husband is happy for you to go with him to his asthma clinic, it can help you to become more involved with his asthma care. You don't say if your husband is already under the care of the asthma nurse or doctor at your practice. If he is, then he needs to talk to them about any concerns he may have about his asthma. It is possible some tests can be carried out at the surgery.

Unfortunately, the actual cause of asthma is not fully understood, but there are trigger factors (see Chapter 2) known to start it off or make it worse. Some of these triggers are known to the individual or family and should be avoided where possible. Unfortunately many people have multiple triggers and it is impossible to avoid them all.

If it seems likely, from talking to the doctor or asthma nurse, that your husband might be allergic to something, allergy tests can be done to confirm this. The most common type is called a skin prick test, in which various substances, or allergens, are pricked into the skin. If the skin reacts and swells up, then the person is probably allergic to that substance. The difficulty is that allergy in the skin is not necessarily the same as allergy in the nose or lungs. In most cases, it is possible to identify the trigger from talking to the person (taking a medical history), and allergy tests often only confirm a fact already known to the sufferer. However, these investigations may help to identify new trigger factors.

Special tests can measure the amount of antibodies (substances produced by the body's immune system) to certain allergens in the blood. If someone has an allergy that is important in causing symptoms, then the levels of antibodies in the blood are very high. The tests are expensive and complicated to interpret.

Some working environments and occupations are known to be linked with asthma and can and do actually **cause** asthma. If you have asthma already, then some working environments can make your asthma worse. The most common jobs associated with occupational asthma are:

- animal handlers
- bakers and pastry workers
- chemical workers
- food processing workers
- nurses
- paint sprayers
- timber workers
- welders.

If your husband finds his asthma is better when he is away from work or on holiday, it is possible that his occupation is making his asthma worse. He should talk to his asthma nurse or doctor about this and, if an occupational trigger is suspected, he must be referred to see a specialist occupational health chest doctor as soon as possible.

**What is the role of the doctor in controlling asthma?**

The doctor probably has the most important role in making sure that the diagnosis of asthma is made correctly and in starting you on the right treatment. Other people become more important in the day-to-day control of the condition. Most important of all is the person with asthma – you! You are the one who has to take the treatment day in and day out, to recognize symptoms of asthma coming on, and to take action to deal with them. Contact with doctors is only a tiny proportion of day-to-day living. This is why it is essential for people with asthma to take an active part in the control of their own condition, so that they are able to lead their lives as fully as possible, unrestricted by their asthma.

Trained asthma nurses play a major part in providing care for people with asthma. These nurses work in hospital asthma clinics, in general practice and in schools. The doctor does retain vital roles in the ongoing management of asthma. These are to:

- prescribe suitable medication, although some nurses and pharmacists are now able to prescribe asthma medicines as well

- follow up people with asthma when they are well

- help people with asthma and their families to monitor their asthma, and to recognize when asthma is going out of control

- treat in cases of emergency.

### What is the role of a practice nurse in the prevention and treatment of asthma?

This depends a great deal on the practice and the individual nurse concerned. Many general practices are now devoting much more time to looking after people with asthma, and the practice nurse usually plays a major role. Often there is a system of shared care between the GP and the nurse but the nurse's role will depend on their knowledge of asthma as well as their training in asthma management. This may range from a fairly minimal role – perhaps recording a patient's peak flow measurements and checking inhaler technique – to a much higher level as is the case with an asthma specialist nurse, who has much more responsibility. In many practices, the role of the asthma nurse includes:

- obtaining a full asthma history

- recording and interpreting peak expiratory flow readings

- confirming the diagnosis of asthma together with the GP

- developing an appropriate asthma treatment and action plan in partnership with the person with asthma and the GP

- demonstrating, teaching and checking inhaler technique

- providing asthma education and counselling to enable someone to manage their asthma

- setting up a well-organized system for regular review of asthma symptoms, lung function tests, asthma medicines and inhaler delivery devices

- being readily available to give advice especially with worsening asthma

- treating acute asthma attacks according to current asthma guidelines.

We do not believe that nurses should be asked to take on this level of responsibility without receiving specialized training. Many practice nurses do have specific asthma training and have developed a high level of expertise. Their aim is to help people maintain optimum control of their own asthma, and to minimize its effect on their lives. As we have said in the previous question, some asthma nurses are also able to prescribe asthma medicines, after special training.

It is important that at least one GP in the practice is also particularly interested in and knowledgeable about asthma. People with asthma will receive the most effective care if there is teamwork and good cooperation between the GP, the asthma nurse and the hospital.

### How do I let my GP know what I want, when he seems to want to be in charge?

You have asked about one of the most important areas in the practice of medicine. Good communication between GPs and their patients is absolutely vital if the best outcome for any long-term problem is to be achieved. Sadly, poor communication occurs far more often than we would like. GPs often fail to understand what the needs of the patients are. People often fail to understand why GPs are worried about them, and how they are trying to treat their asthma (or other problems).

In an ideal situation, your GP or asthma nurse will take care to find out what you expect from the consultation. In asthma, you should be given an opportunity to show how much you know about your asthma, and your feelings about treatment. The GP or asthma nurse can then explain the facts and discuss treatment choices with you in a meaningful way. Following this you can both agree on a treatment or action plan. Unfortunately this does not always happen!

People's expectations are very different. Some visit the GP hoping for a prescription that will cure their problem. Others wish to discuss their health, and then make their own decision on treatment. The GP–patient relationship should be a two-sided one, with both having a say in the treatment plan. Friction usually results from a failure on both sides to communicate clearly. In your own case it may be difficult because your GP believes that he or she knows what the best treatment is. GPs may feel defensive if you have another viewpoint that challenges their own. For example, you may be seeking a cure for asthma while your GP may believe the best course of action is to avoid attacks by taking regular preventive treatment. In your own case think carefully about the points you wish to discuss before you go in to see your GP. Book extra time for your consultation. Try not to leave before you have discussed them! It may help to take your partner or a friend along with you.

Sometimes GPs and patients cannot get along with each other no matter how hard they try. When this happens it may be best to agree to differ, and to change to another doctor.

## *Recognizing uncontrolled asthma – preventing attacks*

**My 'puffer' inhaler doesn't work any more. What is wrong with it?**

We assume that you are using your inhaler (*puffer*) correctly in the first place. If so, there could still be several reasons for this. It could be that the hole through which the medicine is delivered has become blocked with deposits of medicine particles. If you breathe in and out of the inhaler mouth several times before depressing the canister, condensation from your breath can increase the likelihood of it becoming blocked. It is important to clean the inhaler regularly as recommended in the patient information leaflet that comes with your inhaler medicine.

Another more obvious reason for it not to 'work' any more is that it could be empty! It is not always easy to tell how much remains in the canister. Many people learn how to measure this by shaking the canister gently, and getting a feel for how much is left. It is much easier to tell when one of the new CFC-free puffers is empty – they simply stop working! Some inhalers have a counter but do remember to check to see if it is empty!

Sometimes people say (and feel) that their inhaler is not working when in fact there is nothing wrong with it. There are two important explanations for this:

- People may be confused about the type of inhaler they are using – for example confusing a preventer and a reliever. Some people misunderstand the way in which preventers are supposed to help their asthma. A preventer steroid inhaler does not give instant relief and because of this the steroid inhaler may appear not to 'work'.

- More importantly, people sometimes say that their reliever inhaler is not working as well as it usually does, **because their asthma is getting worse**. This is a very important sign of uncontrolled asthma.

### How will I recognize that the asthma treatment is not working, and more or a different treatment is needed?

The two most important clues that you need extra treatment are:

- needing more relief medication
- worsening peak flow readings.

Anyone who needs to take salbutamol ( e.g. Ventolin or Airomir) or terbutaline (Bricanyl) more than once a day should be taking a regular preventer asthma medicine. An increased need for salbutamol or terbutaline warns you that your asthma is out of control and that extra medicine is necessary. This means that:

- a regular preventer asthma medicine is needed if you use the reliever inhaler more than once a day, even if your asthma is usually mild and you normally use it only if you get symptoms

- if you are already using one of the preventer inhaler medicines, and you find that you need to use your reliever inhaler more than once a day, then your dose of preventer inhaler either needs to be increased or other asthma treatment added

- if your reliever inhaler medicine gives relief for less than 4 hours, then this is a sign your asthma is out of control. **If your reliever medicine does not work quickly, or its effects last for less than 4 hours, your asthma is uncontrolled and medical help is needed. Take extra reliever while waiting for help and advice.**

The need for extra doses of the reliever medicines can provide useful information for your doctor or asthma nurse. This information as well as your asthma symptoms and peak flow readings will help your asthma specialists decide if you need a change of treatment such as the addition of a preventer medicine. Peak flow readings that have a wide variation and when plotted on a chart have a 'zig-zag' or 'hills and valley' appearance are another sign that your asthma is out of control.

Needing to use more reliever inhalers, as well as changes in your peak flow readings, will help you to recognize when to:

- adjust your own medication

- call for help.

## Why can asthma attacks be so unpredictable?

Asthma is variable in severity and sometimes asthma attacks are just as unpredictable.

It is difficult for us to explain exactly why sudden attacks occur. Perhaps you are allergic to cats, but you do not always get asthma symptoms when you are in contact with one. Sometimes a combination of triggers or circumstances may spark off an asthma attack. It may be additional triggers such as stress or having just started a cold, moving house or inhaling lots of dust that are the problem. These extra circumstances may be enough to set off an attack when you come into contact with the cat.

More often, asthma **is** predictable, but people are not aware of it. For example, some people continue to go into stables even though the hay and the horses are the triggers for their attacks. Others insist on smoking, even though this makes their asthma worse. By avoiding known personal trigger factors, many 'unpredictable' asthma attacks could be prevented.

If you have an asthma attack, then you need to start urgent treatment yourself. For some people these unpredictable asthma attacks can be very severe and it is important to carry supplies of emergency asthma medicines to use in such a situation.

### How can I prevent an asthma attack?

Most asthma attacks can be prevented, but some cannot. The key to preventing attacks is to avoid your known trigger factors if at all possible, and to recognize your early warning signs. Take extra reliever treatment as soon as possible and call for medical help if this does not work. Most severe attacks can be prevented by these actions. You should discuss your own circumstances and actions with your doctor or asthma nurse.

Important signs of uncontrolled asthma are:

- increased symptoms

- lowered peak expiratory flow readings (PEFs)

- an increase in the gap between the morning and evening readings ('morning dipping')

- PEF readings steadily dropping.

The charts in the section on ***Blowing tests*** later in this chapter show examples of these changes.

### What should I do if my son panics and becomes breathless?

You don't say what age your son is but, if your son panics, try to stay as calm yourself as you can and encourage him to stay calm as well. This is not easy, but the more you panic, the worse he is likely to become. In some children (and indeed some adults), overbreathing brought on by panic or fear of an attack can be almost as distressing as asthma itself. However, it is difficult to be sure that breathlessness is due to overbreathing unless you are very experienced in managing your son's asthma. It is better to treat him as if it is asthma causing the problem.

Firstly, give him high doses of reliever inhaler medicine such as 15–30 puffs of Ventolin Evohaler or Airomir (salbutamol). This action is safe, and will help to open up the airways. If you have a spacer device (Volumatic [now discontinued – Figures 4.14 and 4.15], Nebuhaler [Figure 4.16], Nebuchamber [Figure 4.17], Aerochamber [Figure 4.18], Pocket Chamber [Figure 4.19] or Able Spacer [Figure 4.20]), it is best to give the reliever inhaler using a spacer, giving one puff every 10 seconds. If not, any sort of emergency chamber, such as a paper or plastic cup, or even a paper bag, will do (see Figure 8.1 in Chapter 8). It is better to get a small amount of the medicine into his airways than none at all. It is important that only one puff is squirted into the spacer at a time. In other words, puff once just before he breathes in; wait until he has breathed in four or five times through the spacer and then puff again.

If this does not help within minutes, then it is an emergency situation that needs urgent medical help. If this cannot be obtained from your GP practice, dial 999 so that he can be taken to the nearest casualty (Accident and Emergency) department by ambulance. This will get you and your son to hospital quickly and safely, and the ambulance will also carry oxygen which is essential in the treatment of severe asthma attacks.

If your son has been prescribed prednisolone tablets as part of the treatment for acute asthma, give him the recommended dose as soon as you can, preferably before you go to hospital. These medicines take about 6 hours to work, so it is important to start as soon as possible. Use the dose that has been previously agreed with your doctor – this is usually 20 mg for children aged 2–5 and 30–40 mg for children over 5 years).

**Should I carry an inhaler with me during the day, even if I expect to use it only at both ends of the day?**

This depends on the type of inhaler you are talking about. The preventer inhalers such as Becotide (beclometasone), Alvesco (ciclesonide), Flixotide (fluticasone), Asmanex (mometasone) and Pulmicort (budesonide) are normally prescribed once or twice a day. These are steroid inhalers that do not need to be carried around with you during the day – they will not give you immediate relief from symptoms and so are not used 'on demand'. Two other types of inhaler that may have been prescribed twice a day are Serevent (salmeterol) and Oxis or Foradil (formoterol). These are long-acting relievers, so they do not need to be carried with you.

Short-acting reliever inhalers (e.g. Ventolin, Bricanyl, Airomir, Salamol, salbutamol, terbutaline, Pulvinal [salbutamol]) are for immediate relief of symptoms, and should be kept with you at all times in case they are needed.

# Peak expiratory flow monitoring

### Why do I need to use a peak flow meter?

Because it gives you a lot of information about your asthma! Measuring the peak flow can help to show you when an attack is on the way, how bad the attack is and also when your peak flow readings are better.

The peak flow meter in Figure 5.1 gives a reading (peak expiratory flow or PEF) which tells you how wide open or tight your airways are. The more widely open the airways, the faster air can be blown out of the lungs when you breathe out forcefully, and the higher the PEF reading. Normal PEF readings vary for adult men and women depending on their age, sex, ethnicity and height (**not** weight). During episodes of uncontrolled asthma (exacerbations), the airways become narrowed and the PEF falls.

The PEF will often show a drop in readings a few days before symptoms develop. This helps you to decide when to increase your

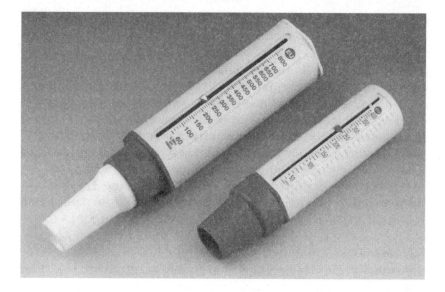

**Figure 5.1** Mini-Wright peak flow meter.

asthma medicines to prevent an attack or episode of uncontrolled asthma. The PEF can also be of help in confirming that your asthma control is good. If your PEF readings are normal for you, and there is very little change from day to day, then your asthma is well controlled.

If you have had an asthma attack, the peak flow readings can help you tell when you are better. Once the readings have got back to normal, it is safe to stop taking emergency medication (steroids and higher doses of inhaled medicines).

**I've got a peak flow meter, but what is a normal reading?**

'Normal' readings are usually shown in a chart inside your peak flow meter box. These readings depend on your age, sex, height and ethnic group, but there is a problem with using them. There is a very wide range of 'normal' readings for any particular person's age, sex, height and ethnicity.

We prefer to use the **best** value achieved by someone instead of using 'normal' PEF values. In other words, each person finds out what their own **'tailor-made normal'** readings are. This reading can be used to tell if the asthma is well controlled or not when compared with day-to-day readings.

There are a few ways to find out your best or personal normal peak flow reading. One way is to keep a chart when you are well. Write down the best of three peak flow readings when you wake up and do the same again in the early evening. Take a few more readings during the day if possible. You can mark these on a chart (Figure 5.2) available from your doctor or asthma nurse, or it may be downloaded from Asthma UK's internet site (see **Appendix**). Alternatively, if you are not happy using graphs, the readings can be written down as we have done in Figure 5.3. Look at the readings and see what the best readings are when you are at your best. It may take some time to establish this, but knowing your personal best peak flow is more accurate than using the graphs.

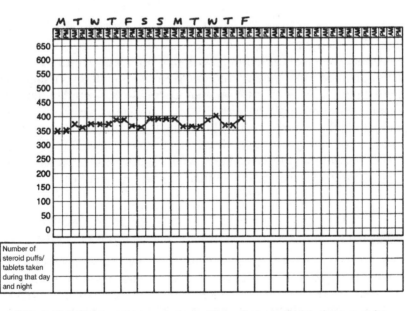

**Figure 5.2** This graph, in a person with well-controlled asthma, can be used to determine the 'best ever' peak expiratory flow (PEF). In this case the readings average around 370, and this could be used as the 'best ever' PEF.

| Day | Morning readings (best of 3) | Evening readings (best of 3) |
|---|---|---|
| Monday 25th | 230 | 200 |
| Tuesday 26th | 300 | 350 |
| Wednesday 27th | 300 | 330 |
| Thursday 28th | 350 | 350 |
| Friday 29th | 330 | 370 |
| Saturday 30th | 320 | 400 |
| Sunday 31st | 350 | 320 |
| Monday 1st | 250 | 250 |
| Tuesday 2nd | 300 | 290 |
| Wednesday 3rd | 250 | 340 |
| Thursday 4th | 280 | 250 |

**Figure 5.3** A peak flow chart where the readings have been written down in a table.

If your asthma is out of control, the readings will change by more than 20% from day to day and morning to evening, and under these circumstances it is difficult to work out what your best reading is. Therefore the ideal time to find out your best reading is when you are well or possibly after taking a short course of steroid tablets for an attack. For example, look at Figure 5.4. The readings are normally about 350; they then drop to 120 during the attack and then return to 350 after taking steroid tablets. This person's 'best PEF' is 350. If there are a few very high readings, while the majority are a bit lower, it is best to use the commonest high reading as your best.

### At what times of day should I record my peak expiratory flow?

The peak flow reading is usually at its lowest in the early hours of the morning and at its highest some time between mid-day and evening. If you record your PEF twice daily before any reliever treatment, this will give you a good record of your asthma control. The best times are in the morning, soon after waking and in the early afternoon. If you cannot do the afternoon readings, then do

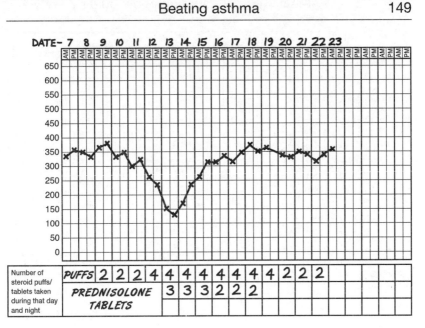

**Figure 5.4** This person's readings are normally about 350, as seen at the start of the chart. They then drop to 120 during the attack and then return to 350 after taking steroid tablets. This person's 'best PEF' is 350.

them during the early evening. Make a note of the best of three blows whenever you take your PEF. Morning readings alone are helpful, but it is really best to do afternoon or evening readings as well, because this shows how your asthma control changes during the day and night.

### How do I do a peak flow chart and how do I know if my asthma is OK?

Your peak expiratory flow (PEF) readings can be written down in a simple number form such as in Figure 5.3. This chart shows that the PEF readings are sometimes very low and at other times much higher. It is not difficult to see that this person's asthma is out of control. There are two key indicators of this. Look at:

- **The highest and the lowest readings.** In this chart the lowest reading is 200 and the highest is 400, which means

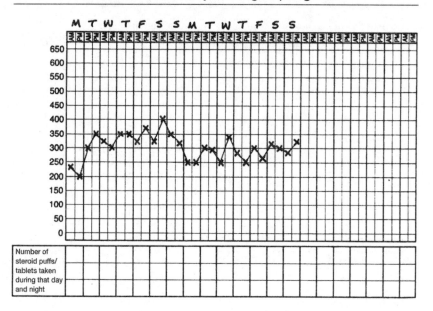

**Figure 5.5** This chart shows a child's readings whose asthma is clearly out of control. The readings vary from morning to evening and from day to day.

that the highest reading is double the lowest. When asthma is well controlled, there should be very little difference between the day-to-day readings or between the morning and evening readings (less than 20%, and usually less than 10%).

- **The difference between the morning and the evening readings on the same days.** In this chart, morning and evening values are almost the same at times and at other times very different. This gives an idea of the variation from morning to night, which is called the *diurnal variation*.

Like many people, you may find that graphs are a lot easier to follow than written down values. The peak flow chart in Figure 5.5 shows the PEF readings in a graph, but they can also be written down in number form as in Figure 5.3.

There are a few things to look for in peak flow graphs. Look at:

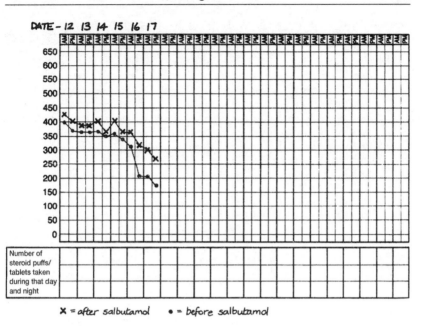

DATE - 12 13 14 15 16 17

X = after salbutamol    • = before salbutamol

**Figure 5.6** The readings before and after relief inhalers (salbutamol) are different, indicating poor asthma control. The sudden drop was a dangerous indication that things were going wrong and this man needed hospital admission.

- **The pattern.** Normal peak flow graph readings should stay roughly the same and be almost level (as in Figure 5.2). The graph in Figure 5.5 shows very uneven lines.

- **The gap between the morning and the evening readings.** In Figure 5.5, on the first Monday they go from 230 to 200. On the next day, Tuesday, they go from 300 to 350. The difference between these readings is 15–20%, indicating that the child's asthma is out of control.

- **The change from day to day.** This is easier to see on the graph in Figure 5.5 than the chart with the numbers in Figure 5.3. For example, the change from the Monday to the Tuesday, and the change from the Sunday to the Monday, are very clear.

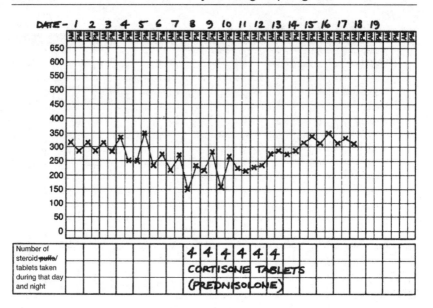

**Figure 5.7** This 7-year-old child's peak flow chart shows increased gap between the morning and evening readings and his response to prednisolone (steroid) tablets. The chart helps to decide when it is safe to stop the steroid tablets once the readings come back to the best levels.

If the reading is dropping way below your best reading, then your asthma is becoming more troublesome. This is the most important use of the peak flow meter – to see how much readings are changing (varying) from morning to evening, and from day to day. Everyone should know their own personal best reading, so that they have a better opportunity to identify when asthma is going out of control, and the risk of an acute attack increases.

### How useful can a peak flow meter be?

A peak flow meter is very useful as it gives an indication of how tight your airways are. When your asthma is well controlled, your twice-daily readings should be almost the same every time they are taken, although the evening reading is usually very slightly higher. The readings should not vary by more than about 20%. An example of a peak flow chart which shows good asthma control is

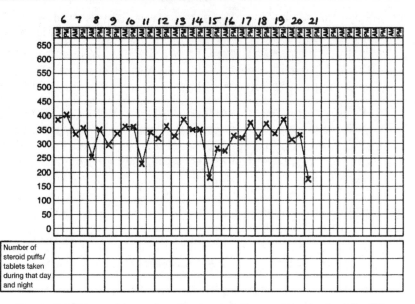

**Figure 5.8** The early morning dips in peak flow on this chart on the 8th, 11th, 15th and 21st of the month were very serious warnings of uncontrolled asthma. This person needed additional treatment, and the doctor was consulted urgently.

shown in Figure 5.2. As discussed in the previous answer, the main indicator that your asthma is uncontrolled is when the readings change a lot from day to day. Figures 5.3–5.5 show PEF readings of poorly controlled asthma.

The charts can be used in a number of ways, but first you need to find out what your normal readings should be (see the earlier question in this section). Once you know your normal readings, the peak flow meter makes it easier to make changes in treatment and to decide whether you should contact your doctor, asthma nurse or the hospital. There are some warning signs that an asthma attack may be coming, which we illustrate here with some examples.

- **If the readings are dropping** (see Figure 5.6). The dots show the readings before relief inhalers (salbutamol) and the 'x's show the reading after relief medication. In this chart the readings dropped slowly but steadily from the 12th to the morning of the 16th. Then suddenly they dropped further on the evening of the 16th through the 17th. This man needed hospital admission on the 16th because his asthma was so bad.

- **If the gap between morning and evening readings is widening** (see Figure 5.7). This 7-year-old child's peak flow chart started off reasonably level. From the 4th of the month, the gap between the morning and evening readings starts to widen. The readings change from 330 to 250 on the 4th, then from 250 to 350 on the 5th. The readings then drop from 270 on the evening of the 7th to 150 the following morning. The wide gap between the readings is a danger sign. This child needed prednisolone tablets (four a day) in addition to more of her usual inhalers to treat the attack.

- **If there are some dips in the readings, in other words some readings are a lot lower than usual** (see Figure 5.8). The early morning dips in peak flow on this chart on the 8th, 11th, 15th and 21st of the month were very serious warnings of uncontrolled asthma. This person needed additional treatment, and the doctor was consulted urgently.

### How do I obtain a peak flow meter?

Peak flow meters (see Figure 5.1) can be obtained on a National Health Sevice prescription in the UK. Your GP or asthma nurse will be able to prescribe one for you. There are several different makes of meter, and your doctor's prescription should state exactly which meter is required.

A peak flow meter will help you monitor and improve your asthma control. Ask your doctor or asthma nurse if you are in doubt about whether you should have a meter; opinions differ over who should have one. Some health professionals believe that all, others that only those with more troublesome asthma – perhaps those who require frequent courses of steroid tablets or who are on high doses of preventer medicine – should have a meter to use at home.

**My child is 3 years old, and on regular asthma treatment. When can he start to use a peak flow meter effectively?**

If your son is only 3 years of age, it is better to monitor asthma symptoms rather than peak flow readings. There is certainly no value in peak flow readings if they are inaccurate and unreliable. Teaching very young children to blow peak flows can cause confusion between the action of breathing in to take their inhaler treatment, and blowing out to record their PEF. If this happens they may not take their treatment effectively. It is better to abandon the peak flow readings until they can easily separate the two actions. Most children are unable to record a reading reliably until they are 5 or 6 years of age. Certainly by the age of 7 they should be able to use a peak flow meter (see Figure 5.1).

Windmill trainer devices are available for the low reading Mini-Wright flow meter and these are quite useful when trying to encourage young children to blow into a peak flow meter.

**Why do peak expiratory flow readings vary so much in the mornings and why do people with asthma have a 'morning dip'?**

In this sense, 'morning dip' is nothing to do with a trip to the local swimming pool! Asthma symptoms do tend to be worse during the early hours of the day, and the PEF is usually at its lowest at this time. This drop in peak flow is called a 'morning dip' (see Figure 5.8). There are many theories about the cause of the morning dip, but no certainty. Possible explanations include posture when asleep, leakage of acid from the gullet into the airways, low body steroid levels during the night, and even low levels of body growth hormone during the night. Many careful research studies have investigated this problem, but have not yet provided definitive (definite) answers. The readings are usually highest sometime between mid-day and the early evening.

In practical terms, the size of the morning dip gives a good idea of how poorly controlled the asthma is. Treatment aims to remove, or at least minimize, the morning dip and in people whose asthma is well controlled we see little or no dip in the morning PEF reading.

This is why it is best to make at least two measurements of PEF during each 24 hours to assess the amount of morning dip because it will vary from person to person.

Some people have apparently well-controlled asthma, but still experience large morning dips in their PEF. The addition of a long-acting bronchodilator medicine such as salmeterol (Serevent) or formoterol (Oxis or Foradil) may help to reduce the morning dip, and is often an effective addition to preventer treatment.

**I have two peak flow meters, one for home and one for my bag. If I use both at the same time I get different readings. For example, if one reads 530 litres per minute, the other reads 480 litres per minute. Does this matter?**

It does matter because no two meters are exactly the same. There are several types of peak flow meter, and several different manufacturers. One is shown in Figure 5.1. Different meters often give readings that vary by 10% or more, even if they are of the same type and make. These differences may be small, but can be important and confusing for people with asthma, as well as for the doctors and nurses caring for them. It can be misleading to compare readings from home (on a prescribed meter) with the doctor's own meter in the surgery or outpatient clinic.

The ideal approach is to use the same meter consistently on each occasion. Since peak flow meters are available on prescription in the National Health Service, it is possible for nearly everyone to have one, and to take one's own peak flow meter when attending any clinic. If this is not practicable, then at least be aware that there can be an important difference between meters. In your own case, if you do find it necessary to have two meters, then the difference between the two should be consistent, and as long as you are aware of the variation you can make allowances for it.

The readings on peak flow meters are measured in *litres per minute*. This is explained in the *Glossary*.

# *Written action plans for asthma*

## What is an asthma action plan?

Asthma action plans are also known as 'self-management plans' and have been used increasingly in the past few years. The title is rather grand, but an action plan is simply an agreement between you and your doctor or asthma nurse about the steps you can take to deal with your symptoms before calling for medical help. In this way you become much more involved in the day-to-day control of your condition, and can respond to changing needs for treatment.

These sorts of agreements have existed for years but the emphasis has changed recently in two important ways:

- It is much more likely that plans will be written down. A range of cards, charts and booklets has been developed to enable the plan to be written down clearly.

- Secondly, in most cases (except for young children), PEF readings will form an important part of the plan, so that at certain peak flow levels, changes in treatment are triggered. These levels will vary from person to person depending on a number of factors. For example; your plan might say that you should start a course of prednisolone tablets if your PEF reading drops below 250, when it is normally between 480 and 520. In this case, you would start this course of treatment without needing to see your doctor or asthma nurse first. **The figures and treatments we give here are only examples, and you should not use them to manage your own asthma. Discuss a similar plan with your own doctor or asthma nurse.**

Some plans are quite complex, with a number of steps that may be taken, depending on changes in symptoms and PEF readings. Others are much more simple, for example saying, 'If your PEF reading falls below 50% of your best reading, take 2–20 puffs of your reliever inhaler, and see your doctor or asthma nurse urgently.'

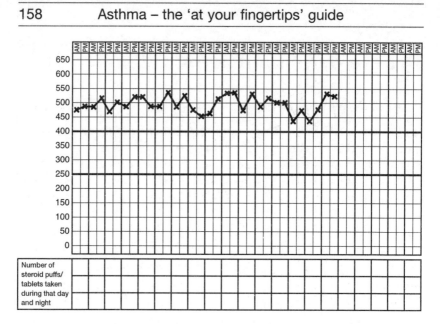

**Figure 5.9** This chart shows action lines drawn at 80% and 50% of this person's best PEF.

Research has shown that asthma action plans work better if they:

- are written down

- use the personal best readings rather than general 'normal' readings

- have recommendations for the use of both inhaled and oral steroids.

### How do I work out the percentages on the action (self-management) plans?

Calculating a percentage target for PEF is a useful way of guarding against uncontrolled asthma. The idea is to discover the best peak flow that you can achieve, and then to use this as a 'benchmark' or standard, against which action levels can be calculated.

If you take PEF readings regularly, when well and completely free of symptoms, you will soon establish what your own best reading is. Action levels for increasing treatment are calculated at

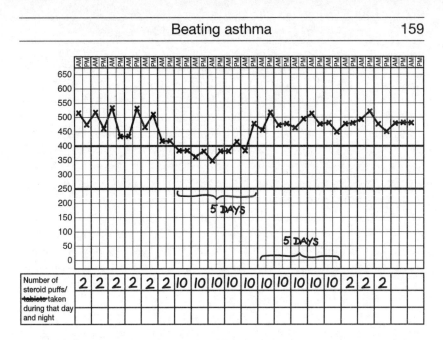

**Figure 5.10** If the readings drop towards the bottom line, in this case at 50% of best, then decisive action is needed. This person has followed his action plan, which advised him to increase his preventer inhaler to five times the usual dose, 10 puffs a day, until he was better.

certain percentages of this. A quick way to work out the percentages is to use a calculator and multiply your best readings by 0.1 for 10%, 0.2 for 20%, 0.3 for 30% and so on. This is all probably best explained by an example, using the chart shown in Figure 5.9. In this case, the person involved has a best PEF reading of 500 when he first consulted. Two action levels are calculated.

1. An 80% level (multiply the best reading of 500 by 0.8):

$$500 \times 0.8 = 400$$

2. A 50% level (multiply the best reading of 500 by 0.5):

$$500 \times 0.5 = 250$$

Two lines are drawn on a peak flow chart at these 80% and 50% levels, and used as guidelines. If the PEF readings stay above the top line (80% of best) then the asthma is well controlled, and treatment does not need to be changed. If the readings drop towards the top line, usual treatment needs to be increased (see Figure 5.10). If the readings drop towards the bottom line, in this case at 50% of best, then immediate action is needed.

Extra doses of relief medication should be taken straight away, and the dose of inhaled steroid medicine needs to be increased. There is no absolute amount the dose should be increased by, and we advise that the dose should be increased to a level where the asthma is controlled. If this means increasing the usual dose by 4- or 5-fold, this is acceptable if it helps you regain control of your asthma. The dose is then reduced once the symptoms and peak flow come under control. Prednisolone tablets are probably needed when the readings continue to go down or reach the second line at 50% of best – in this example, at 250 litres/min. Urgent medical advice will be needed at this point.

These two levels of action (80% and 50% of best readings) are probably the two used most commonly, but the great advantage of such action plans is that they can be made to suit the individual. Many doctors and asthma nurses add a third level and advise patients to call for emergency help if the readings drop below 33% of their best. It is essential for you and your doctor or asthma nurse to decide on the most suitable action plan for you. The important first step for such action plans is to know your own 'personal best' PEF.

### How long should I continue to take my preventers at the higher dose?

The peak flow chart may be helpful in answering this question; when the readings return to the 'best level', lower the dose. Some people find their asthma follows a set pattern, where they know how long their asthma episodes usually last for and therefore when it is safe to reduce the dose towards their previous level. Another practical way of reducing the dose is to count how many days it took from the time your PEF readings dropped below the line, up until the day when they reached your previous best levels. Then simply carry on taking the higher dose for the same number of days. As an example, look at the chart in Figure 5.10 where the normal (best ever) peak flow is about 500. Two action lines have been drawn at 400 (80%) and 250 (50%). This person increased his inhaled steroid dose from two to five puffs in the morning and evening. He continued at this dose until the readings returned to the normal level. He then counted how many days it took him to get to this point (5 days). Then he continued at the increased dose for the same number of days, i.e. for another 5 days.

## Holiday plans

An agreed holiday action plan to deal with an emergency is also extremely helpful, and here is an example (see also Figure 8.5 in Chapter 8).

If your PEF drops below 50% of your normal or best previous levels there are a number of things you can do:

- Try to remain calm.

- Take multiple doses of your reliever inhaler (either Bricanyl – generic name terbutaline; or Ventolin Evohaler – generic name salbutamol; or another salbutamol inhaler). In an emergency take one puff or dose every 10 seconds until you feel better (you may need 15–30 puffs).

- Take a dose of prednisolone tablets. Before going away on holiday agree with your doctor or asthma nurse the dose you should take in an emergency. Continue taking daily prednisolone tablets until the attack is over.

- If you are not getting better with the reliever medicine, see a doctor urgently; call an ambulance, or the emergency services.

- See your own doctor or asthma nurse as soon as possible when you get home.

This is merely an example; you should agree individual medicines and doses with your own doctor or asthma nurse.

Always remember to make sure you have adequate health insurance if you are going abroad for your holiday. It can be very expensive if you do not have enough insurance cover.

# *Altering and changing treatment*

**Am I allowed to alter my treatment, or should my doctor always do this?**

Doctors and nurses who have an interest in asthma aim to help their patients become expert in managing their own asthma. Thus, a major role for the health professional is to enable people with asthma to take care of their asthma themselves, while consulting with them regularly to reinforce this independence. This means that a clear action plan must be agreed. This will usually include the following information:

- Extra asthma medication will be needed if you are likely to be exposed to known asthma triggers.

- Common symptoms of asthma will lead to a need for an increase in asthma medicines. If this helps, the dose will be continued according to the action plan.

- It is usual to continue at the increased dose for a while until recovery takes place. The length of time will vary from person to person and between different episodes of asthma.

- There are no fixed rules, only guidelines. In these circumstances the use of peak flow readings and charts may be very helpful.

- If the increased asthma medicine fails to help there need to be guidelines as to when to obtain urgent medical help.

In medical jargon this type of approach is called 'guided self-management'. This is a type of asthma action plan. It means that you can alter your treatment with changing symptoms or changing PEF readings according to your agreed plan.

Consult your doctor or asthma nurse if problems arise and your self-treatment is not working. There is a section on action plans (also known as self-management plans) earlier in this chapter.

## How long do I need to take my medicine for?

This depends on your age and other factors. Asthma is generally a lifelong condition. People do not outgrow their asthmatic tendency, although the disease often goes quiet for a while, perhaps for many years. This is called the remission phase of asthma. Unfortunately, however, it will sometimes flare up again in later life after exposure to an obvious trigger; more often it flares up for no apparent reason.

Asthma can be unpredictable and because of this you may be helped best by taking continuous treatment aimed at preventing the inflammation process in the airways. This treatment may be needed for a long time – possibly even years – after your symptoms have 'gone quiet'. If your asthma has gone into a truly prolonged remission, then your treatment could be reduced or even stopped. Ideally you should use peak flow readings for guidance when reducing or stopping treatment. Treatment should be resumed if your symptoms come back.

In adults, asthma treatment is usually for life. However, some adults get only short episodes of asthma and once these have cleared up completely, with little variation of the PEF, it is worth reducing or stopping the treatment. The use of a peak flow chart in this situation is very helpful in deciding whether treatment should be resumed.

## Do I have to stay on Becotide forever?

Like the answer to the previous question, this depends mainly on your age and the severity of your asthma. Adults usually need to remain on preventive treatment for a number of years, often for life.

## If prescribed asthma medicines are taken regularly, is it ever possible to cut down the dose and, in time, give the medicines up altogether?

Yes, it is possible. As a rule of thumb, the longer your asthma symptoms have been kept under good control by treatment, the less likely it is that symptoms will come back if you reduce your treatment. In treating asthma, most health professionals will try to help you control your symptoms with the lowest possible dose of medication. So, when your symptoms are well controlled, your asthma medicines should be reduced, and even stopped if this is possible. The dose can then be increased or restarted if your symptoms start again. Nobody knows the answer with certainty. Some people feel that symptoms should be controlled for a year before treatment is reduced ('stepped down'). Others believe that dosages can be reduced much sooner.

Regular checking with a peak flow meter makes it easier to adjust your treatment. If you have few symptoms and your peak flow readings vary only slightly from morning to evening, then it is probably safe to reduce your asthma medicines. Discuss this question with your doctor or asthma nurse to see if your asthma medicines can be reduced.

**Can we decrease our son's asthma medicines? He has just had his 7th birthday, and has been well for 2 months.**

Possibly, but discuss it with your doctor or asthma nurse because the dosage of medicine may be just right to control your son's symptoms. Two months without problems is very encouraging, but it may be a little soon to adjust his treatment; between 3 to 6 months is preferable.

For children, most doctors would advise treatment for at least a year or at least while symptoms remain. If the child is able to use a peak flow meter, daily peak flow readings will make sure that all is well. Treatment might be stopped and restarted only if the readings continue to vary by more than 20%. Some children may not have any further trouble from their asthma, but the family should be aware that it could flare up suddenly, even after a number of symptom-free years. This is why it is so important to have a written action plan and enough asthma medicine when you go on holiday.

In our view, once children have started asthma treatment, they should continue taking medication for at least a few months after symptoms have resolved. The main factor is the initial severity of the asthma. If after a period of treatment, the asthma is very mild and there are few symptoms or attacks, then therapy might be stopped. In older children, this is best done with the help of a peak flow chart which provides early warning of deteriorating asthma. It may be better to stop asthma treatment after the coughs and colds season because they are the main asthma triggers in children.

We believe peak flow meter readings are very helpful. A chart will show whether it is safe to decrease your son's asthma medicines. A level peak flow chart such as the one in Figure 5.2 would indicate that the asthma is well controlled. The graph is almost a straight line. In this case you could try reducing his medicine, and then monitor the peak flow readings. If the readings stay level, and there are no symptoms, then it is safe to continue on the lower dose. If the readings do begin to vary, then the control of asthma is being lost, and the previous dose should be taken again.

As a rule of thumb readings should not go up or down by more than 20%. The formula to calculate this change (variation) is:

$$\frac{\text{Highest} - \text{lowest reading}}{\text{Highest}} \times 100 = \% \text{ change in peak flow}$$

If the change is greater than 20% then the variation is too high and his asthma is out of control. For example: if the highest reading during the week is 400 and the lowest is 300, the peak flow variation is therefore 25%, and would indicate that the asthma is quite badly out of control.

As long as the peak flow readings do not go up or down by more than 20% then it is safe to stay on the lower dose. In a few more months it may be possible to make another reduction in the treatment. As mentioned in an earlier question it may be better to make any reductions to your son's asthma treatment after the coughs and colds season, because they are the main asthma trigger in children. However, bear in mind that the end of the coughs and colds season also heralds the hay fever season, if this sort of allergy is a problem for him.

**Is it better for me to put up with my asthma, and not take any asthma medicines?**

No, and if putting up with asthma means that you are having symptoms then the answer is definitely no. The presence of asthma symptoms means the presence of inflammation of the airways. Asthma inflammation is an ongoing process which may damage the lungs. The presence of inflammation makes the asthma more liable to flare up and result in an attack. We feel that people whose asthma is causing them regular symptoms should be taking regular anti-asthma medicines, which reduce the underlying inflammation. Such preventer medicines include those described in Chapter 4: beclometasone (e.g. Becotide), budesonide (e.g. Pulmicort), fluticasone (Flixotide), mometasone (Asmanex), ciclesonide (Alvesco). Nedocromil sodium (Tilade) and sodium cromoglicate (Intal) are used less often now because inhaled steroids usually work better; however, they may be appropriate for some people.

**When can I stop my steroids after an attack?**

The best way to decide this is with the help of a peak flow meter and a daily chart. Most health professionals now accept that people with asthma can follow an action plan for self-management once one has been agreed between those involved. There is a section on asthma action plans earlier in this chapter, and information on managing emergencies is also provided in Chapter 8. The basic guidelines for such a plan are as follows.

- The usual PEF reading is taken as the normal or best reading. If you have your own meter, you will usually have a good idea of your normal readings.

- When the peak expiratory flow drops below 30–40% of the normal reading, a course of steroid tablets will normally be offered. The dose is usually 20 mg/day for children aged 2–5 years; 30–40 mg/day for children over 5 years and 30–60 mg/day in adults.

- The tablets are continued at this daily dose until the peak

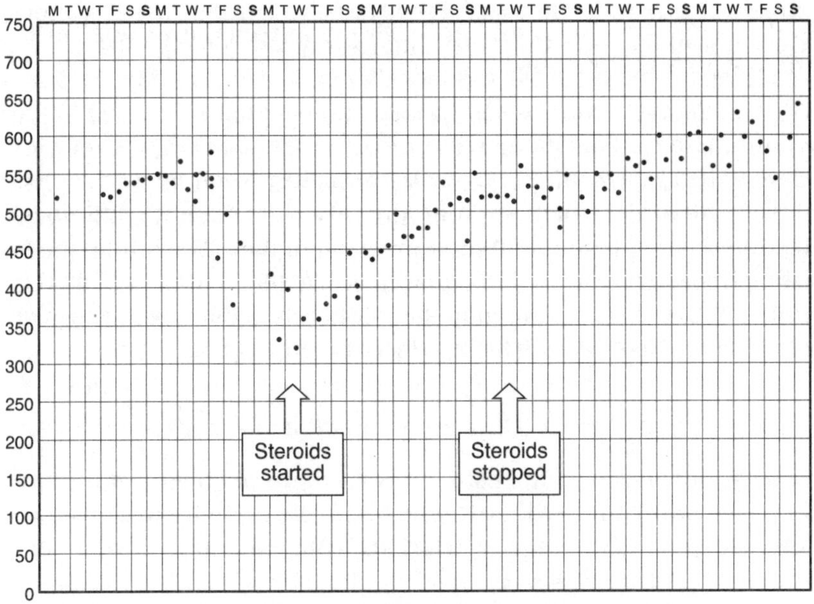

**Figure 5.11** This person knew from his chart that steroid tablets were needed when his peak flows dropped dangerously from his normal readings. He was also able to tell when it was safe to stop them when his peak flows were almost back to the usual best readings.

flow reaches your normal value. It is important to keep taking these tablets until a good response has been achieved. The time this takes is different for everyone. A peak flow chart is very helpful in deciding when it is safe to stop taking these tablets; this is usually when the readings have got back to the 'best ever' and stayed the same for a few days. In young children 3 days' treatment is often sufficient to gain control of asthma symptoms.

- See your asthma nurse or doctor frequently after an attack until you are better and you will soon learn how to deal with any future asthma attacks.

An example may help to explain all this more clearly. Figure 5.11 shows the chart of a person who has managed to treat an asthma attack successfully. He was keeping a daily chart, his usual readings were about 500 litres/minute, and he started getting wheezy. His readings dropped to 320 and he saw his doctor that day. A course of prednisolone tablets was started and his doctor advised him to continue taking his inhaled steroid. He saw the doctor every few days until 11 days after starting the steroids, when he was advised it was safe to stop them, because the peak flow readings had almost returned to his best readings. This was the first attack this person had experienced and a plan was agreed with the doctor. This real-life example from a patient helps to demonstrate why a peak flow chart helps in treating asthma attacks.

### How can I recognize that my treatment is working?

You can recognize your treatment is working when your symptoms improve and your peak flow chart has returned towards normal. The use of a daily peak flow chart is particularly helpful when new treatment has been started or when the dose of existing treatment is increased. Signs of improvement on the chart are:

- your readings are fairly constant, without variation from morning to evening, and from day to day

- your readings are improving towards your normal or 'best' values.

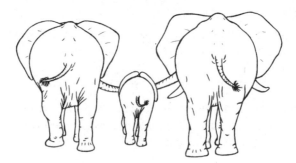

**Personal action plan – things you might wish to discuss
with your doctor or asthma nurse**

Once you have read through this chapter, there may be a number
of things you might wish to discuss with your doctor or asthma
nurse. These may include:

- asking for a prescription for a peak flow meter and learning
  how to keep a peak flow chart

- finding out what triggers your asthma and how to prevent
  exposure to these triggers

- finding out how often you should attend the surgery for
  asthma check-ups

- checking that you are on the right asthma medicines and
  whether the dose needs to be adjusted

- agreeing an asthma action plan for yourself (or your child),
  and ensuring you have the right asthma medicines

- knowing what to do if you have a severe asthma attack

- finding out how your doctor's practice works and how you:

  - arrange a routine check-up

  - obtain a repeat prescription

  - get help in an emergency.

# 6
# Living with asthma

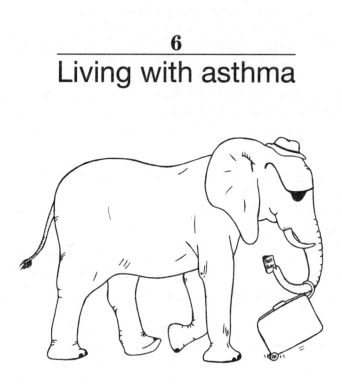

In this chapter you will learn about:

- how to cope with asthma

- why asthma does not need to rule your life

- asthma and work

- asthma and food allergy

- physical fitness and asthma

- holidays and what you can do to help prevent asthma attacks.

While it is important to try to avoid things that make your asthma worse, asthma does not have to rule your life. This chapter deals with some of those very practical questions which concern people with asthma and about which they have asked us. As with the other chapters there are several sections, but all deal with different aspects of the environment in which we live. There is certain controversy about why there has been an increase in asthma over the past 25 years. It seems that there has been a significant increase in the number of children with asthma, and some people think that this is due to changes in our environment, particularly the effects of pollution.

We have been asked questions by a number of women as to why asthma may get worse during periods or just before them. This is a well-recognized problem and some women with asthma do have problems related to their pregnancy or to their periods. Clearly the body sex hormones have some influence over asthma because hormonal changes occur not only in pregnancy and periods but also during puberty.

Asthma in the workplace was given great prominence during 1991 when a woman won industrial compensation from her employers because of the adverse effects on her asthma of cigarette smoke in her work environment. More recently experts in the UK have made recommendations for the prevention and treatment of occupational asthma. In addition, they have tried to raise awareness among health professional colleagues of particular occupations that are more likely to cause occupational asthma.

Holidays should be a time for you to enjoy yourself, rather than thinking about your asthma. Forward planning can prevent problems occurring from acute asthma attacks in faraway places.

Following the enormous changes to the National Health Service during the last 15 years there has been concern about the costs of treatment for asthma. There is considerable pressure on health professionals to reduce prescribing costs wherever possible. However, at the time of writing this edition of our book, we know of no circumstances where the correct treatment for asthma has been justifiably withheld on the grounds of cost. Good asthma treatments are not cheap, but if they improve short- and long-term health of people with asthma, and prevent expensive hospital admissions, then their prescription costs will be fully justified.

# Everyday life

### Can someone's asthma be affected by their social background?

There is some evidence that social background can have an effect on asthma. Some studies have shown that asthma is more common in families with one or two children compared with larger families. Another finding suggests that children from higher socioeconomic groups are more prone to asthma. Why this happens is not entirely clear at present, but research has come up with one interesting suggestion. This shows that the youngest children in large families seem more likely to catch lots of colds and respiratory infections in early childhood from their older brothers and sisters. These infections seem to boost their immune systems, so that they are less likely to develop allergic conditions like hay fever. Children in small families seem less likely to catch these early infections, but more likely to suffer from allergic conditions, which we know are strongly associated with asthma.

Another important factor in the social background is whether there are smokers within the family. It is a fact that smoking is more common in poorer socioeconomic groups. Smoking by mothers with a history of asthma makes it more likely her baby will have asthma; smoking during pregnancy results in smaller babies with smaller airways, making them more susceptible to wheezing illnesses. We know that children who are exposed to smoke in early childhood are more likely to have wheezing illnesses (but not necessarily more asthma). The key message is that smoking is bad, both for your health and for that of your children.

### Why is my asthma at its worst when I carry heavy shopping?

Carrying shopping is a strenuous activity and any strenuous exercise or activity may trigger asthma symptoms. If exercise makes

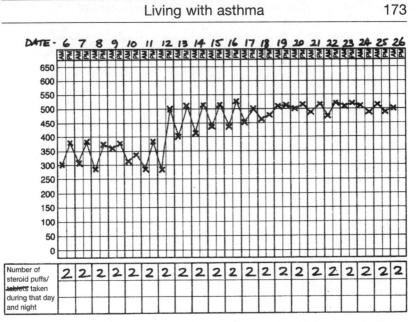

**Figure 6.1** This is an example of a chart where the readings gradually improve after treatment.

your asthma worse only on occasions such as this, you could prevent it by taking an extra dose of reliever medication just before the activity in question. However, if this is a more regular problem and your asthma gets bad every time you exercise, then you probably need to take more preventer medication or to start preventer treatment, if you are not already on it. There are sections on actions plans for self-management in Chapter 5 and on treatment in Chapter 4. You probably need more preventer medicine treatment if you have to take your reliever medicine more than three times a week for asthma symptoms. Talk to your doctor or asthma nurse about this.

We make no apology for repeating the advice that a daily symptom diary chart can help in finding the right dose of treatment to prevent symptoms (see Figure 3.1 in Chapter 3). If your morning and evening readings show a wide difference (more than 20%), then you should follow your agreed action plan. This will probably include increasing your preventer medication (inhaled steroid) by four or five times and, of course, taking more reliever medication

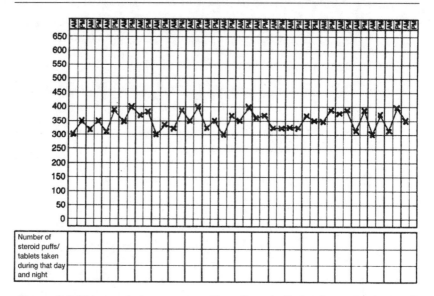

**Figure 6.2** This graph, in a person with well-controlled asthma, can be used to determine the 'best ever' peak flow (PEF). In this case the readings average around 370, and this could be used as the 'best ever' PEF.

as needed, until your readings no longer vary by so much from morning to evening (or from day to day). In addition, depending on the agreed action plan with your doctor or asthma nurse, you might also start a short course of steroid tablets. Once your asthma is controlled, the readings on your chart will be almost the same each day (in other words, they will not vary much from day to day) and therefore the graph will appear almost flat. Figure 6.1 shows an example of a chart where the readings gradually improve after treatment; Figure 6.2 shows the chart of someone with well-controlled asthma.

### Why is asthma often bad at night?

This is another good and simple question with a complex answer! In short, nobody knows for sure. There are various theories, which have been the subject of much interest and research.

Waking at night with asthma is very common. It means a disrupted sleep so you probably feel tired in the morning. A bad asthma attack at night can also be very frightening. Some of the favoured explanations for asthma problems at night include:

- how you lie when you are asleep
- dust and house dust mites in the bedding triggering asthma symptoms
- low levels of certain body hormones at night (particularly cortisone and growth hormone)
- increased acid production by the stomach
- changes in air and body temperature
- asthma medicines taken earlier in the day not having a long enough effect.

This is quite a list and, although no doubt all play some part, most have been ruled out by research as major causes by themselves.

Perhaps the most important explanation is that a change takes place in the body's natural rhythms during the night. All of us (whether or not we have asthma) have an individual lung function pattern during a 24-hour period. Some people may have high PEF readings early in the afternoon, while others might be high during the morning. On average, though, the best (highest) readings are between mid-day and 1400. In poorly controlled asthma, the early morning readings are usually much lower, and breathing can worsen dramatically at this time. Remember that, if your asthma wakes you up, it is out of control! The low readings of early morning match the low point for hormones that are produced by the body, and the two are probably connected. We still have much to learn about asthma at night but one thing we can say for sure is that good day-time control leads to improvements in night-time asthma.

**I sometimes wheeze when I go near a dog, or it is very dusty. Is this an allergy, or asthma?**

It is probably both – asthma symptoms triggered by your allergy. Dogs and dust are both important potential triggers of asthma. The allergic reaction to the dog or dust may make you wheeze and cause an asthma attack if it is not treated promptly so that it settles down. As well as triggering asthma there may be other signs of allergy, especially skin itching, runny nose and sneezing, and itchy eyes.

### Why do I wheeze when I go into a warm house from the cold outside?

Changes of temperature are responsible for making you wheeze, particularly when your airways are irritable and sensitive. A sharp change in temperature may set off an asthma attack. It may be that your symptoms begin outside in the cold, but become worse when you get indoors. Cold air is a well-known trigger of asthma symptoms, and going from a warm house to the open air in the winter frequently makes people cough and wheeze. Other allergens such as dusts, moulds or animal hairs may also trigger your symptoms as you move into the indoor environment.

### Why do I feel uncomfortable in gas central heating and feel better when cool?

You are not alone in experiencing this problem, and many people have noticed that their asthma seems to get worse in centrally heated houses. There are several possibilities. House dust mites are a common trigger of allergic asthma and we know that warm, centrally heated homes are ideal conditions for the house dust mite population, which increase in great quantities in this warmth. If there are any gas fumes from the boiler, these could also increase your discomfort. Even during winter months when the central heating is needed most, it is a good idea to have some outside air circulating in the house. Open gas fires may also make asthma worse.

A further possibility is that, if your asthma is not very well controlled, a change of air temperature from the cool outside to the warm inside can trigger symptoms. Finally, it is worth remembering that, if anyone in the home smokes, it is more likely to cause problems than the central heating!

**At the beginning of the winter months when the central
heating is switched on, my nasal passages feel very tickly.
What can I do about it?**

There are two likely explanations for these symptoms. One is
allergy to the house dust mite, and the other is the onset of cold
winter weather. This condition is called rhinitis. Many people with
asthma also suffer from rhinitis.

In allergic rhinitis the lining of the nasal passages reacts to
trigger factors (allergens), in just the same way as the lining
of the airways does in asthma. The reaction may be a tickly
sensation, a feeling of being blocked or even a runny nose
with frequent sneezing. There are many possible allergens,
but in your case house dust mite allergy is the most likely
cause. Another well-known allergen is grass pollens, which
cause hay fever. Although the house dust mite causes problems
throughout the year, the numbers are at their highest during
the early winter months. Switching on the central heating gives
a boost to their numbers by raising the temperature. Warm,
centrally heated houses with fitted carpets and curtains
provide almost the perfect environment for house dust mite
numbers to multiply!

Ironically, cold weather is another trigger factor for rhinitis. This
is not a true allergy, but is usually called vasomotor rhinitis. Cold
air causes a reaction in the lining of the nose, with results similar
to those of allergy.

If your rhinitis is very troublesome, we suggest that you talk to
your doctor, asthma nurse or pharmacist about it. There are several
highly effective treatments, and most of them are available over
the pharmacist's counter.

**Is it all right to buy a cough medicine for my tickly cough
when I have inhalers for my asthma?**

Asthma symptoms such as tickly coughs may develop into full-
blown asthma attacks if they are not treated properly. We would
not recommend you buying cough medicines and we would go so
far as to say it is often a waste of money.

There is really no place for cough medicines in the treatment of asthma since there is little evidence that they help the coughing caused by asthma or, for that matter, chest infections. Your tickly cough is almost certainly a sign that the asthma is not properly controlled by the treatment that you are already taking, and it is very important to recognize and appreciate this. The use of cough medicines may provide some temporary relief, but this could delay starting effective anti-asthma treatment. Rather than use cough medicines you should increase your inhaler use, or talk to your doctor or asthma nurse about how you can adjust your treatment.

If you do want to try something to soothe your tickly cough, home remedies such as lemon and honey and hot water are just as effective and a lot cheaper than over-the-counter cough medicines!

### Can I give blood?

In general, anyone who requires regular prescribed medicines cannot be accepted as a blood donor. This applies to everyone who takes regular medicines, not just those with asthma. We do not recommend that you stop your regular asthma medicines as your asthma could go out of control. If you need to take only occasional reliever treatment such as Ventolin or Bricanyl, you will be accepted as a blood donor. These are the guidelines of the National Blood Service for people with asthma, but they may be interpreted differently by the various transfusion centres. It would be advisable to contact your local transfusion centre yourself in order to confirm our advice regarding your suitability as a blood donor.

### Are people with asthma more at risk than other people when given a general anaesthetic?

The answer to this is no – providing that your asthma is well controlled. Your lungs need to be in as good a condition as possible and the airways unrestricted. If you know that you are going to be given an anaesthetic, then it would be well worth you doing a series of peak flow measurements, if possible, for about 2 weeks beforehand. (See the sections covering peak expiratory flow in Chapters 3 and 5 for more details about this.) You can then check that your asthma is well controlled. If this is not the case, make sure that you see your doctor or asthma nurse as soon as possible, rather than just before your operation.

It is obviously important that anaesthetists know that any patient has asthma, so that they can take any extra steps that might be necessary. In some hospitals the anaesthetist will ask those with asthma to use a nebulizer before they are given the anaesthetic. This ensures that the airways are as wide open as possible. Fortunately the anaesthetist is in a very good position to check and put right any breathing problems that might occur during an anaesthetic.

People with severe asthma and those with other chronic lung conditions are at much greater risk when given an anaesthetic than someone whose asthma is well controlled. Nowadays the range of operations that can be performed under a local anaesthetic is much greater, and so people who are at increased anaesthetic risk because of lung problems are given general anaesthetics less often.

**I have asthma. Is it safe for me to have an operation?**

There is no reason why you, or anyone else who has asthma, should not have an operation. Many surgical operations require a general anaesthetic, and we have discussed this in detail in the previous question.

It is important to continue your asthma treatment after the operation. Unfortunately, some hospitals take away the patient's own inhaler device and substitute it with a different type. If this happens to you, ask the doctor why your asthma medicines have been changed. Ask the doctor or nurse to check that you are able to use any new inhaler device correctly. Some hospitals use only the pressurized metered dose inhalers but not everyone is able to use this device and careful instruction is needed. If you are not happy with any new asthma treatment, speak to your GP or asthma nurse when you leave hospital.

**Will asthma affect my son's future regarding getting insurance?**

This depends on the severity of his asthma, the type of insurance he needs and also whether he takes the medicines prescribed by his health professional. Sickness benefit and life insurance may be more difficult to obtain at usual premiums than endowment insurance. People with the most severe asthma and those requiring long-term treatment are likely to receive insurance quotations that will cost more than usual premiums: in other words, the premium is loaded. However, some companies are more sympathetic than others, and there are a number of different companies to choose from. It is best to shop around for the best buy. An independent insurance broker, not tied to any one company, is in a good position to do this on your son's behalf.

For every application for insurance, the GP is asked to provide a medical report for the insurance company. Provided the applicant has signed a consent form, the GP will disclose relevant medical information to the insurance company. This information may help or hinder the person's chances of obtaining a low premium. For example, someone who fails to take regular treatment for asthma despite medical advice may be loaded with a higher premium, as a result of the disclosure of this information. On the other hand, someone who is careful, and who follows a treatment plan and attends regularly for check-ups, may get a lower premium from the company.

Your son is entitled to see the report before it is sent to the company. He may ask for it to be altered if he disagrees with it, but the doctor is obliged to tell the insurance company that alterations have been made, or if information has been withheld.

**What about keeping pets? I have asthma and my child wants a pet cat – do I go ahead and get him one?**

This is an interesting question, and unfortunately we cannot give a definitive answer. If you have asthma and you are sensitive to certain animals, your asthma is likely to be worse if they live in your home. Having pets to which you (or your child) are allergic is not a good idea.

There has been a lot of debate over the years on the so-called 'hygiene hypothesis'. Some scientists believe that children who have early contact with more infections and allergens are less likely to get asthma and other allergic diseases. There is some evidence that supports this idea; however, there is also evidence that doesn't! Children who live on farms seem less likely to get allergies but the research has not proved this beyond doubt. The way this works is that when people are in contact with allergens (substances that cause allergy, like cats, dogs, pollen, dust mites or certain infections), they develop antibodies to them. The antibodies can then work either to protect against disease or actually cause disease if the person is exposed to larger quantities of those allergens. Whether a child develops asthma depends on two things: whether the child is allergic, and how much allergen they come in contact with.

At the time of writing this book, we are unclear whether pet ownership definitely protects children against developing asthma or whether pets are a cause of asthma. From the current research information we would not advise getting rid of animals if children are born into pet-owning homes. If the child (or someone else in the family) develops an allergy, you will need to decide whether to find a new home for the family pet. It would be worth discussing this with a health professional.

Whether you go out and get a pet after the child is born is another question which we would prefer not to answer!

## *Smoking*

**I have heard that girls and women suffer more from asthma than men if they smoke – is this true?**

There is some research evidence that there are differences in asthma and the effects of smoking between men and women. Women seem to be at greater risk of developing asthma if they have smoked. This is very important because the tobacco industry seem to target young women with their advertising campaigns.

Before puberty, asthma is more common in boys than girls. After puberty more women suffer from asthma, and there are many possible reasons for this. Smoking may be one of them. Lung function in women who have smoked or who have been exposed to other people's smoke is found to be worse than in men. Women who have smoked are likely to have more 'twitchy' airways compared with men, and are also more likely to be admitted to hospital for lung problems.

### I have heard that smoking doesn't affect asthma – is that true?

No! This may be some sort of folklore that goes back to the days when asthma cigarettes (which contained herbs, not nicotine and tar) were sold as treatments for the condition. This was a very early form of inhaled treatment!

There is very strong evidence that asthma is made worse in the presence of cigarette smoke. This applies particularly to children, who may have to suffer in smoky atmospheres through no fault of their own. A UK female asthma sufferer recently won industrial compensation because she suffered the harmful effects of involuntary or passive smoking. This has heightened public appreciation of the problem. Increasingly, workplaces are becoming non-smoking areas, because the harmful effects of involuntary (passive) smoking are now known.

Perhaps even more worrying is the evidence that an increase in smoking among pregnant women and mothers is causing the development of asthma symptoms in their children later on in childhood.

### How can I stop my husband smoking in front of the children?

Parents who smoke are putting their children's health at risk, both in the short and long term. Often people are simply unaware of the risks posed by passive smoking. Perhaps if you can convince your husband of these facts he might be prepared to smoke away from areas of direct contact with your children.

There is increasing evidence for the harmful effects of cigarette smoke on children's asthma. We know that:

- infants exposed to passive cigarette smoke suffer from more wheezing illness during the first year of life than infants who are not exposed

- lung growth and lung function in children whose parents smoke are not as good as in those whose parents do not smoke

- cigarette smoke is a trigger factor for asthma attacks.

The problem is particularly bad for children with asthma whose parent(s) or relatives smoke at home. Research suggests that children whose mothers smoke suffer most, and that this is far worse for those children who are at home all day rather than away at school or nursery. The main risk factor seems to be the length of time the child spends with a smoker.

We are sure you will be aware that the issue of smoking can sometimes be a cause of friction in the family! If your husband wants to stop smoking, encourage him to go and seek professional help. Many practice nurses are very experienced in counselling people about smoking cessation. Your local pharmacist is also likely to be a source of help as well.

### How can I ask people in my work environment to stop smoking?

It is not easy to impose a complete ban on smoking at work. There is no doubt that when smokers and non-smokers share the same room, non-smokers cannot avoid inhaling some of the tobacco smoke as they breathe – this is called involuntary or passive smoking. We know that exposure to tobacco smoke can cause discomfort and irritation, particularly to those who already have a chest problem such as asthma. The tobacco smoke concerned is mainly the 'sidestream' smoke from burning cigarettes, cigars or pipe tobacco, but there is also some smoke exhaled by smokers. Tobacco smoke contains various substances that trigger unpleasant asthma symptoms.

At work, consultations should take place with all the people involved. Imposing measures to control involuntary or passive smoking can lead to resentment among smokers, and problems in enforcing the non-smoking rule. Limiting or preventing smoking by an agreed and carefully implemented policy is more likely to:

- improve employee morale

- reduce arguments between smokers and non-smokers

- reduce time lost through sickness

- reduce cleaning bills!

Perhaps you could suggest that smoking is limited to certain areas of your workplace. This is a perfectly reasonable request, and you should not feel that you are being difficult or demanding. Perhaps you could join other non-smokers at your place of work and act together in making your request. After all, it is not only people with asthma who are keen to see this sort of control on places for smoking.

**I am 19 and I have asthma. I enjoy going to pubs and clubs with my friends at university but the next day I find that my asthma is really bad. I am sure it is the smoky atmosphere. What can I do?**

You are probably right about the smoky atmosphere as smoke is known to make asthma worse. We suggest you make an appointment to have your asthma checked by your doctor or asthma nurse. They will want to know if you get asthma symptoms at any other times, what they are and how often you need to take your blue inhaler. They will also do some simple peak flow tests and check how you use your inhaler device. All these things will help them to assess your asthma control. This will help them decide whether you are on the right asthma treatment, or whether you need to have extra treatment.

If you are already on a preventer inhaler make sure you remember to take it regularly not just when you have symptoms.

A common mistake is to take the preventer inhaler only when unwell rather than regularly. Try using your blue inhaler before you go to the pubs or clubs – that may be sufficient to help relax your airways and prevent you having problems. If all else fails it may be worth trying to find somewhere to socialize that is less smoky. Fortunately, the law is changing and there will be more smoke-free areas in the future, especially where food is served.

# Sex, periods, pregnancy and the menopause

## Sex

**Asthma seems to interfere with my sex life – why?**

Although asthma is such a common condition it is not a frequent cause of sexual difficulties. However, if asthma does occur during sex it can cause problems. Symptoms can be brought on by:

- exertion, which can prevented by the use of a reliever medicine (such as salbutamol or terbutaline) before intercourse

- movement in bed, which can sometimes cause large amounts of allergens to be released from the bed clothes, triggering wheezing

- allergy to a partner's semen (sperm), although this is very rare. An allergy to latex condoms is also rare and can cause a generalized allergic reaction, which may include asthma. This can happen suddenly, with catastrophic results. This is called an *anaphylactic attack* which could be life threatening. This can happen up to 6 hours later (also called a late allergic reaction). Latex-free condoms are available but anyone allergic to latex should consult an allergy specialist.

As far as we are aware asthma medicines do not affect sexual desire or responses.

**Does the oral contraceptive pill weaken the effects of reliever or preventer inhalers?**

No! The contraceptive pill may even be a good form of treatment for asthma in some women. If your asthma gets worse about 2 weeks before periods start, we suggest you record your peak flow and discuss the results with your doctor or asthma nurse. Oral contraceptive therapy may be useful in your case. If the peak flow drops at the time of ovulation (usually about 14 days before the next period), the contraceptive pill may prevent asthma attacks by blocking ovulation.

If you are taking a pill with a high dose of oestrogen, you should check your peak flow regularly because high doses of oestrogen therapy may be associated with a drop in peak flow in women with asthma.

## Periods

**Could my periods have anything to do with my asthma?**

Quite possibly, as it is likely that the menstrual cycle has an effect on asthma in many women. Research has shown that, in some women, asthma gets worse during the week before a period (menstruation). This link between getting asthma symptoms before periods seems to be more of a problem in some women with severe or poorly controlled asthma. We know that such women can have severe asthma attacks around the time of menstruation. Research has reported a drop in peak expiratory flow (PEF) and increase in symptoms at the time of menstruation in as many as one in three women with asthma. Remembering to take your preventer asthma medicines regularly will help to keep your asthma under control.

If this is the case with you, you would benefit by monitoring your peak flow either regularly or in the week leading up to your period. Any changes in peak flow will alert you to take extra asthma medicines when needed. An asthma action plan based on peak flow readings will be useful. This can also help to identify when to seek advice for poorly controlled asthma. (See the section on peak expiratory flow in Chapters 3 and 5 and *Written action plans for asthma* in Chapter 5). The best way to do this is to keep a peak flow diary of your readings for at least 3 months to see if there is a regular pattern of a consistent fall in PEF around or before your period. If so, then that is strong evidence to support your suspicions and it would be sensible to increase your preventer treatment during the week before falls in peak flow are expected, to see if this helps. If it does not help you should go and see your asthma nurse or doctor.

Many women take pain killers and anti-inflammatory tablets for period pain, and this is another possible cause of poor control of your asthma during periods. Aspirin and similar anti-inflammatory drugs such as Nurofen (ibuprofen) and Ponstan (mefenamic acid) are frequently used for period pains. They are all members of a large group of medicines known as non-steroidal anti-inflammatory drugs (NSAIDs) and they can cause symptoms of asthma, particularly in those people who are allergic or intolerant to aspirin. These pain relief medicines are best avoided if you have asthma. If you need to take regular medicines for period pains check with your doctor, asthma nurse or pharmacist what else may be suitable for you.

**Once a month I've ended up in hospital, back on steroids, and being nebulized. This is because of my periods. Why?**

There is strong research evidence that demonstrates a link between asthma and periods (see previous question). Exactly how female hormones affect asthma is not known, but the changing levels of oestrogen and progesterone during the monthly cycle are likely to be the cause. Some women report that their asthma becomes worse around the time of menstruation, but it is a minority. You are doubly unfortunate in having such severe problems.

In the rare cases of life-threatening attacks before periods (premenstrually), the problem does not always improve even with high-dose steroid asthma treatment. Some women find that progesterone hormone therapy (given by injection) is helpful. Others find the oral contraceptive pill helps to prevent the sudden change in hormone levels with subsequent improvement in asthma control. Discussion between a respiratory specialist and a gynaecologist is essential to plan the best possible treatment options with you. There are further options, but it would be best to discuss these in detail with the experts.

## Pregnancy

### What effect does being pregnant tend to have on asthma?

Pregnancy has a variable effect on asthma. Research has shown that for some women their asthma actually improves during pregnancy. During pregnancy, you have high levels of oestrogen in your blood, and for some women this may make asthma worse. Around 40% of women require more treatment to control their asthma during pregnancy, around 40% keep to the same treatment and around 20% actually need less. Recent studies have shown that the health of a newborn baby is unaffected by whether or not the mother has asthma.

Any risk for the baby during pregnancy, comes from uncontrolled asthma and severe acute attacks. It is important therefore to try to prevent this from happening. All pregnant women with asthma should have regular check-ups with the doctor or asthma nurse to make sure that their asthma is well controlled. This might mean increasing or changing medication.

Acute asthma attacks may cause a shortage of oxygen for both the mother and her growing baby and this may be dangerous. It may result in smaller babies and even stillbirth in severe asthma attacks, although the latter is extremely rare. The preventer asthma medicines (e.g. Becotide, Pulmicort, Flixotide, Qvar, Beclazone and Pulvinal [beclometasone] are safe in pregnancy and are important in preventing asthma attacks (see the next question). We have less experience using the newer inhaled steroids of Asmanex ( mometasone) and Alvesco ( ciclesonide) in pregnancy.

**I've just been told I am pregnant – can I still take my medication?**

Yes, your medication can and should be taken, provided you are taking it through the inhaled route. In the first 3 months of pregnancy, the general rule is to take no medicines by mouth (i.e. tablets or syrup) unless they are really necessary. Your doctor or asthma nurse can advise you about this.

Asthma medicines that are taken by inhaler are safe during all stages of pregnancy. If you are already taking montelukast tablets for asthma, it is safe for you to continue taking them, but they should not be started during pregnancy. If asthma is poorly controlled or you have an asthma attack, a short course of steroid tablets may be necessary. It is better to take a short course of steroid tablets than risk harming the baby through uncontrolled asthma.

It is very important for you to try and control your asthma during your pregnancy. If you have severe asthma attacks, the main risk to your baby is that he or she may be born underweight. In a very severe asthma attack, there is a tiny but real risk of infant death.

During pregnancy, regular peak flow monitoring and more frequent asthma check-ups will alert both you and your health professionals if your asthma is getting worse.

**Will I get breathing difficulties in labour?**

As long as your asthma is well controlled, your breathing should be no different from that of any other woman in labour. At the end of pregnancy, the womb (uterus) takes up a lot of extra space in the abdomen. This causes pressure, which pushes the diaphragm upwards and 'squeezes' the lungs. In late pregnancy and in labour, this results in breathing being slightly more difficult. If your asthma is bad, then an extra strain will be placed on your breathing, and you may notice some difficulties. Talk to your health professional if you are worried about your asthma control in the later stages of your pregnancy.

The anxiety and excitement that occur when labour begins may result in you forgetting to take your asthma inhalers. You may even leave them at home in the rush to get to hospital! It is a good idea to pack an extra inhaler in your maternity suitcase to avoid this. You can also help prevent breathing problems in labour by using the breathing exercises that you have been taught at antenatal classes, and by taking your asthma medication regularly.

### Is it OK for me to breastfeed while taking Ventolin and Becotide inhalers?

Yes! If you can breastfeed, this is the best possible start you can give your baby.

In usual doses, Ventolin and Becotide asthma inhaler medicines are absorbed in such miniscule amounts into your system that any traces will be almost undetectable in breast milk. If you use a spacer device to take your asthma medicines (a Volumatic [now discontinued, Figures 4.14 and 4.15] for Becotide and Flixotide; an Aerochamber [Figure 4.18]; an Able Spacer [Figure 4.20]; or a pocket chamber [Figure 4.19], which fits all metered dose inhaler devices), this will reduce even further the amounts of the medicines that are swallowed and absorbed. This removes the chance of these medicines appearing in your breast milk.

### Will breastfeeding reduce the likelihood of my baby developing asthma, or its severity?

Yes, and it will also offer protection against developing eczema. There is new research evidence that full breastfeeding during the first 4 months of life results in fewer children having asthma at the age of 4 years. Partial breastfeeding (mixed bottle and breast) does offer some protection but not as good as in the case of full breastfeeding. Other research suggests that the children who are breastfed may get less severe asthma than those who are not.

In addition, it seems that children who are exposed to cigarette smoke are better off if they are breastfed. While we are **not** suggesting that it is OK to continue to smoke, it seems that, if you cannot stop smoking, your child's asthma may not be as severe if your baby has been breastfed. In addition, the evidence is quite strong that breastfeeding protects against the development of atopic eczema when there is a family history of the condition. Breastfeeding needs to continue for around 6 months to reduce the chances of the baby becoming allergic to cow's milk, and then developing eczema.

Overall, we believe that, with regard to asthma and allergies, it is much better if babies are breastfed if at all possible, particularly where one or both parents are atopic or have asthma and also if the child is exposed to smoke in the home.

## Menopause

**I am going through the menopause and my doctor has put me on hormone tablets because I am having lots of problems. Will it make my asthma worse?**

Although lung function declines with increasing age, it is difficult to be certain what happens to asthma as women go through the change of life (menopause). There is some evidence that increased twitchiness within the airways is associated with this treatment, and that means an increased risk of asthma. We cannot be certain whether hormone replacement treatment will have any effect on your asthma. You don't say how severe or how well controlled your asthma is, but the better controlled your asthma is, the less likely you are to be troubled by the change or hormone replacement treatment.

Make sure to take your treatment as discussed with your doctor or asthma nurse and have your asthma checked regularly.

**I have read that steroid tablets cause brittle bones. Will my asthma inhalers cause the same problems?**

Osteoporosis, or thinning of the bones, is a side effect of long-term steroid tablets, but it also occurs as a result of hormonal changes that happen with increasing age: decreasing oestrogen levels in women and decreasing testosterone levels in men. An increased life span and decreasing hormone levels also increase the likelihood of bone (especially hip) fractures. A family history of osteoporosis is also a risk factor for osteoporosis.

If you have difficult asthma and take steroid tablets regularly, you are likely to experience side effects from the tablets. Your inhalers are unlikely to have any effect on your bones if you are on less than 800 µg/day of inhaled steroid. If you are using higher doses or having more than 4 weeks of treatment each year with oral steroid tablets, then your bone density could be affected.

We recommend that you continue to take your asthma treatment, but go and talk to your doctor or asthma nurse about your concerns. It may be possible to reduce the dosage without loss of asthma control. They may also be able to arrange for you to have a special test to check for osteoporosis (called bone densitometry).

**I am on steroid inhalers for my asthma. Is there anything I can do to help protect my bones?**

There are several ways to promote healthy bones. They are:

- weight-bearing exercise (walking, for example)
- stopping smoking if you are a smoker
- keeping alcohol levels below recommended maximums
- having a diet rich in calcium (lots of dairy products).

If you are on less than 800 µg/day of inhaled steroid, then the risks of bone thinning from your asthma treatment is small. If your asthma is well controlled, go and talk to your asthma nurse or doctor to see if it is possible to reduce your asthma treatment. It is often possible to reduce treatment without loss of asthma control.

# *Work*

**How do different working conditions (e.g. air conditioning, smoky rooms, etc.) affect different people with asthma?**

There are a number of working conditions that can have an effect on asthma. The type of work you do may be as important as your working conditions. Types of work that may affect asthma include working with:

- animals
- certain spices (e.g. mustard)
- dusts and fumes (e.g open gas fires and gas cookers). See also Chapter 2.

Adequate ventilation in the work place helps to reduce problems. As far as working conditions are concerned, anything that pollutes the air can make asthma worse. Cigarette smoke is the biggest hazard. Air conditioning or heating may recirculate polluted air and increase problems rather than improve them. Fan air central heating may even cause spreading of virus infections (colds), which aggravate asthma. Many employers now realize the risk posed to the health of their employees by smoky environments, and they have banned or restricted smoking in the workplace. We welcome this, and hope it will become more widespread. If you believe there may be a problem with your own workplace, discuss it with your occupational health service if you have one, or possibly your union representative.

**What is occupational asthma?**

There are two types of occupational asthma. One is where asthma starts for the first time in adulthood, and is caused by repeated exposure to substances in the workplace. Most people with this type of asthma develop an allergy to the substance. The second is where someone already has asthma but it becomes worse at work. This is called 'work-aggravated asthma'.

If your asthma consistently improves at weekends, or on days away from work, such as holiday times, you may have occupational asthma and you should be referred to a specialist in this field. Your doctor or asthma nurse may ask you to keep a peak flow diary chart every 4 hours over the period during which you are waiting to see the specialist. You will need to do these peak flow readings when you are at work and at home. If your readings are better when away from work, this will support a diagnosis of occupational asthma.

### Are there occupations I will have to avoid?

Anyone with asthma should avoid occupations that are known either to cause asthma or to make it worse. Occupational asthma is caused by exposure to certain substances and the development of allergy to those substances. Occupational rhinitis (runny, itchy or blocked nose with sneezing) often develops before occupational asthma.

There are a number of occupations in the UK known to cause asthma in previously healthy people. The Health and Safety Executive and the TUC (Trades Union Congress) have published leaflets on occupational asthma, for employees, employers and for health professionals. The British Occupational Health Research Foundation has produced guidelines to help general practices identify both occupational asthma and rhinitis (see addresses in *Appendix*).

Asthma UK has published a workplace charter to highlight the issues of occupational asthma, with the aim of reducing the impact of asthma in the workplace. They have also developed guidelines for employers, to help them make the work environment asthma-friendly (see *Appendix*).

Occupational asthma is an important condition. Asthma may take anything from days to years to develop, after initial exposure to the work trigger. It is the only potentially curable form of asthma provided it is diagnosed early enough and you no longer work within the environment where the occupational trigger is present. It may not clear up even when there is no longer exposure to the responsible substance. If you are working with any of the substances listed below, and you get rhinitis or asthma, it is important to mention this when you see your doctor or asthma nurse. Substances known to cause occupational asthma include those in the box.

There are other occupational causes of asthma. If you suspect that your work may be responsible for your asthma, you should consult your doctor or asthma nurse to help you decide if you should be referred to an occupational specialist. This is important from the point of view of your treatment and future work. People who have developed occupational asthma after working with certain substances may be eligible for industrial compensation.

---

### Substances that may cause asthma in the workplace

- Flour, grain and coffee beans

- Adhesives – in particular the isocyanates used in the manufacture of polyurethane spray paints and surface lacquers – and epoxy resin hardening agents

- Wood dusts, especially hardwoods (cabinet makers are more likely to develop occupational asthma than general builders)

- Soldering flux (containing colophony or ammonium chloride)

- Animals and insects (laboratory workers and farmers)

- Latex (health professionals in particular are at risk)

- Drug manufacture – e.g. cimetidine and certain antibiotics

- Aldehydes (health professionals whose work involves sterilizing instruments)

- Dyes such as carmine

- Metals – aluminium, cobalt, chrome, nickel, platinum salts and stainless steel

- Proteolytic enzymes – in baking, meat tenderizing and detergent manufacture

---

**I have just started a new job in a bakery and my asthma has got worse. Why is this?**

Asthma that gets worse at work, or 'work-aggravated asthma', is not uncommon. There are a number of occupations that can make asthma worse and baking is one of these (see the longer answer to the previous question). You should really ask your doctor or asthma nurse to refer you to a specialist in occupational medicine. They might ask you to do a peak flow chart with readings every 4 hours (at and away from work) for several weeks to try to see if you do have occupational asthma. Doing this while waiting for the appointment can help save time once you see the specialist.

**Will asthma affect my son's future regarding employment?**

With regard to employment, there is a small chance that a history of asthma may cause problems for young adults seeking work. However, people with asthma are just as well qualified as those without, and should stand an equal chance of being employed. Ill-informed employers who believe that they are anxious (or 'nervous') people are discriminating against them unfairly.

Certain occupations or conditions in the workplace could have a bad effect on your son's asthma. Any job that involves close contact with dust, sprays, fumes or poor air quality should be avoided wherever possible, as should occupations where there is contact with any of the substances listed earlier in this section.

Ideally, your son's working environment should be free of cigarette smoke but we realize that it is not always possible to choose your workplace. If he gets a job with a large organization, he should be able to get help from the occupational health department or union representative in improving his working environment.

**My son would like to join either one of the services, like
the police, or even join the Armed Forces. However, he
has asthma and wonders whether he will be eligible for
this type of job.**

Possibly. People with asthma no longer face a ban on joining the
police or fire service under legislation that came into force in
October 2004. They are now included within the Disability
Discrimination Act 1995 and as a result, people with asthma will
be assessed on an individual basis.

The Ambulance Service does employ people with asthma,
provided they meet the requirements of the DVLA (Group 2)
requirements. These include: 'any condition which causes excessive
daytime/awake time sleepiness'. Therefore if your son's asthma
keeps him awake at night, he would not be suitable for this work.
However, being able to work in the front line as a driver or
paramedic will depend on the severity of his asthma. An ambulance
paramedic may be exposed to air pollution and smoke when
attending an incident; therefore it is very important to take
preventer medication regularly if prescribed.

There are potential difficulties for people with asthma who wish
to join the Armed Services. The Army will not accept anyone who
has asthma at the time of applying, or who has had the need for
asthma treatment in the previous 4 years. All Army entrants with
a past history of asthma must have been completely off all anti-
asthma medication for at least 4 years prior to recruitment. There
are no exceptions. Any applicant who has been clear of asthma for
4 years will be assessed by the service specialist who makes the
final decision. Anyone who fails to disclose important medical
information may be dismissed from the service. It is worth bearing
in mind that asthma may remit (go quiet for a number of years),
but may come back at a later date. Someone joining the Army may
be exposed to gases and other triggers, which may make the asthma
return. This is one reason why the Army is very cautious about
asthma. The Royal Navy has a similar policy but the Royal Air Force
does not accept people with asthma.

# *Holidays*

### Does travel cause any discomfort to people with asthma?

Asthma should not normally cause any particular problems during travel. One of the main risks is having an asthma attack and being caught off guard when away from home. This is much more important than any risk associated with the travel itself.

Any circumstances that cause a shortage of oxygen may increase respiratory symptoms and cause discomfort. A holiday where the altitude is above 6000–7000 feet may cause discomfort even for people who do not have asthma, but clearly would be potentially problematic for those with symptoms. So enjoy your trip! It shouldn't cause problems but it is worth planning carefully.

If you take a holiday in the UK it is possible to register as a temporary resident with a local National Health Service GP. It is the easiest and best way to get help unless you are unlucky enough to suffer a serious attack, when urgent transfer to an Accident and Emergency department is indicated. (See Chapter 8 on *Emergencies* for more about when to go straight to hospital.)

All GPs deal with many people with asthma, and so will be experienced in the management of uncontrolled asthma. If you do need to be referred to hospital for severe asthma, then the local GP will know the arrangements for getting help quickly from the local specialist.

If you are travelling abroad, the arrangements for emergency medical care are much more variable, and it is worth finding out about them before you travel. All travel companies and travel agents provide details on emergency medical arrangements for their clients. Make sure that you have adequate health insurance cover when travelling abroad.

### I am going on holiday, and don't want to take my inhalers with me. Is that all right?

No, it isn't! We will assume you are taking both preventer and reliever inhalers, so let's discuss them separately and we will try to give you reasons why you should take both of them on holiday with you.

It is really important that, if your doctor or asthma nurse has prescribed a preventer inhaler for you, you should use it on a regular basis, even if you are fit and well and have no current asthma symptoms. Not using your inhalers means your asthma could get worse and go out of control and could ruin your holiday. Your reliever inhaler is equally important and you should take it with you on holiday, keeping it with you at all times.

If you have an asthma action plan (see Chapter 5), and this has been agreed, take an emergency asthma pack (which includes a short course of steroid tablets) with you whenever you go away, in case of an asthma attack. Travelling to different parts of the country (or the world) may expose you to different asthma triggers. As a result your asthma may deteriorate even if it is normally well controlled.

### I am going on holiday, by air, and I need to take oxygen with me. How do I arrange this?

If you have been prescribed oxygen you do need to disclose this when you book with the airline. The airline medical department will issue you with an appropriate form, which needs to be filled in by you and your doctor. The airline will need to know about your medical condition and in particular how much oxygen you need. The airline's Medical Officer will then let you know if you can travel with them and whether they can provide you with oxygen. All the airlines have their own policies on the cost of supplying oxygen and you will need to take this into consideration when planning your holiday.

You will also need to make arrangements with the airline, well in advance of the trip, for oxygen to be available for you at your destination.

### Will flying affect my inhalers?

Flying will not adversely affect your inhalers and all types of inhaler are safe to use in aircraft. Keep them with you in the cabin rather than pack them in your luggage in the hold of the aircraft. Inhalers should not be exposed to extremes of temperature because it may affect how they work.

If your inhaler is a pressurized canister device, it should be at room temperature when you use it – if it feels cold to the touch then warm it in your hands before use. Cold inhalers may not dispense the correct dose of medicine. Reservoir dry powder devices (such as Clickhalers, Pulvinal, Turbohalers and Twisthalers – see Figures 4.8, 4.10–4.13 in Chapter 4) may be affected by changes in humidity and extremes of temperature.

**My inhaler is pressurized. The airline regulations say that I cannot carry it in my luggage so what can I do? What if I need to use it during the flight?**

Although the regulations may state this, airlines do recognize that people with asthma need to take pressurized inhalers with them on their travels. It is preferable and safer for you to carry your treatment with you in your cabin hand luggage because you have the medication available if you need it. If your luggage goes missing you could lose your inhalers as well! Some airlines, including British Airways, carry their own emergency asthma treatment on some of their flights.

**Can I get my usual inhaler in other countries?**

Some of the newer inhaler devices may be more difficult to obtain than the traditional 'puffers' or aerosol inhalers, which are widely available throughout the world. Most asthma inhaler medicines are available in countries in Western Europe, USA, Canada, Australia and New Zealand with a doctor's prescription. In an emergency, you could probably get a reliever inhaler over the counter as you can in the UK. The formulation, strength and brand name of the medicine might vary slightly from country to country. In the USA you may be able to obtain your usual asthma medicines, but not always. They may have different names and dose strengths and you will need to have them prescribed by a doctor or nurse prescriber. In many countries of South-East Asia you can buy medicines from a pharmacy without a prescription. Make sure that you know exactly what you want, and always check that the medicine is in date and has not been opened or tampered with.

Medical information departments of the major pharmaceutical companies will be able to tell you which of their products are available, in which countries, and under what names. Unless you are away for a long time, we suggest that you always take enough of your inhalers with you if you go abroad. Take at least one spare with you in case you lose the one you are using, and take any necessary emergency treatment with you, in case you have an acute asthma attack.

## Will going skiing make my asthma worse?

In our experience most people with asthma who take to the ski slopes have very few problems. If, however, your asthma is triggered particularly by cold air and exercise you should be aware of this, and be prepared. These days most ski resorts have an abundance of ski lifts so the struggle up the slopes is not particularly strenuous. Altitude may be a problem and some ski resorts in Colorado in the USA, such as Breckenridge (10 000 feet) or Vail (7000–8000 feet) are very high. The USA is becoming increasingly popular for European skiers because of the more reliable snow conditions.

At these high altitudes, the temperature can sometimes drop to as low as –10 to –25°C, particularly with wind chill factor. If it is very cold, this may affect your pressurized canister inhaler. In our experience the new types of aerosol propellant can block at altitude. Washing the canister holder and drying it thoroughly may clear the blockage. Test a couple of doses to make sure your inhaler is working again. In some cases a dry powder device may be better. When it is very cold, it is sensible to take a dose of your reliever before you go out and exercise on the slopes.

Get yourself fit before you go skiing. Taking strenuous activity when you are not used to it is unwise. Any increase in exertional symptoms may be due to lack of conditioning rather than your asthma!

A great advantage of going to a ski resort is that the house dust mite does not survive at altitude because it is colder and humidity is low. If you are sensitive to the mite, your asthma may be better when you are skiing than when you are at home, but it is likely to take weeks rather than days to see any beneficial effect.

Take adequate supplies of your asthma treatment with you and do remember to take out sufficient medical insurance cover. Asthma UK has identified an insurance company that should help people with asthma to obtain better insurance cover at more competitive rates. If you are having problems obtaining insurance cover because of your asthma, check the Asthma UK website for further information or contact their Adviceline by phone for advice (see *Appendix*).

As with any holiday, do make sure you know exactly what to do if an asthma attack occurs. Emergency asthma care and skiing injuries can be costly without adequate insurance cover.

**If I do not normally suffer from 'exercise' asthma, will altitude affect me more than someone who doesn't have asthma?**

At high altitudes, the air is colder and thinner (less oxygen available), and in the winter months it is much colder. Conditions like these affect everyone and may cause light-headedness, nausea and swelling of the feet. This is well recognized as 'altitude sickness' or 'mountain sickness'. If your asthma is well controlled, you should be no worse off than someone without asthma. However, cold air is a well-known trigger for asthma. We can't predict whether you will develop mountain sickness but, if your asthma is severe or uncontrolled, you are more likely to have problems.

On the plus side, the house dust mite cannot survive at high altitudes (see previous question), and this is one of the main reasons why clear mountain air, as in the Alps, can be so beneficial for people with asthma.

If you are planning to go to high altitudes, i.e. above 5000 feet, then you should take extra care to prevent attacks. Try to ensure your asthma is well controlled before you travel. If your peak flow readings are not up to your usual best, it would be sensible to increase the amount of inhaler treatment you take until they are. If you have concerns, speak with your doctor or asthma nurse before travelling.

Once you have arrived at your destination, avoid strenuous exercise until your body has had a chance to get used to the altitude changes. It takes a number of weeks to become fully adapted to very high altitudes, but the first few days are most difficult. Light-headedness and nausea are signs of shortage of oxygen. Extra asthma medicines and rest are advisable if this happens. In extreme cases you may need to come down the mountain to lower heights to recover.

### Will Customs take away my medicines?

In most countries of the world there should be no problems about carrying your usual medicines with you. When you are travelling, take a letter on official letterhead paper from your doctor or practice to confirm that any medicines you carry are prescribed for your personal use. This does not guarantee that Customs will not confiscate your medication in countries that are 'off the beaten track'. If you are in any doubts about the country you propose to visit, we suggest you check with the relevant embassy before you go. Embassy websites are worth checking, though they are not always up to date.

### What precautions should my young children take on school trips and holidays?

They should take enough medication to last for the time they are going to be away. They should be encouraged to take their asthma medicines regularly, and their teachers should be aware of their asthma treatment plan. Give the school a written action plan, which explains when to worry, what the medicines are, and when they should be taken. Also give them a peak flow meter if appropriate.

Your children need to know that they should call the teacher if they start getting symptoms (or if their peak flow rate starts to

drop), especially if this happens at night. They should be reassured
that there is no shame in calling for help if their asthma goes out
of control. They (and the teacher) should also know that they
should take extra medication according to their action plan, when
needed.

For emergencies while away from home make sure that the
teacher has access to a spare reliever inhaler (salbutamol, Ventolin,
terbutaline or Bricanyl), a short course of prednisolone tablets and
a peak flow meter (if appropriate). A written plan helps to explain
the use of these to the teacher, or adult in charge. All of this
information can be written on one of the children's asthma cards
available from Asthma UK. These are available to the medical
profession and the public through Asthma UK. The address is given
in the *Appendix*.

Asthma UK have recently produced a leaflet called *After your
child's asthma attack* and it may be helpful for the teacher to have
a copy of this.

# *Sport*

### Can I participate in any sporting activities?

If your asthma is well controlled you should certainly be able to
play any sports, even if they are very energetic. It is important
though that you receive, and take, the right treatment to prevent
your symptoms from occurring. Most people with asthma are not
restricted in any way in spite of their condition. There are many
sportsmen and women who have asthma and it has not stopped
them from representing their country or, for that matter, even
becoming gold medallists! Paul Scholes, Paula Radcliffe and Karen
Pickering are three international sporting stars who have asthma.

### Is there any harm in doing regular exercise, or can this actually improve my asthma?

Regular exercise will do you no harm providing your asthma is well
controlled. In fact regular exercise of some sort is good for all of

us. Studies carried out to try to find out if regular exercise improves asthma have only shown that overall fitness improves. Improved fitness results in improved lung function and improved wellbeing. This is not quite the same as 'improving asthma'. However, we have had reports from our own patients that, if they do regular exercise, they get fewer problems with their asthma.

**Why does swimming help people with asthma?**

There are two main reasons for this. Firstly, exercise of any type helps to build up stamina and strength. Swimming does this for most of the muscles in the body, but in particular for those which help with breathing. Strengthening your breathing muscles helps to fight asthma attacks when they happen. Stronger breathing muscles also give you a better chance of controlling your breathing at times of difficulty.

Secondly, exercise in a warm moist atmosphere seems to be much less likely to cause symptoms than the same amount of effort given to exercising in cold dry air. Humidity in the air around a swimming pool helps counter the tendency to get asthma with physical exercise. However, chlorine that is used to keep the pool clean may trigger asthma symptoms. If this is a problem it is sensible to take a couple of puffs of your reliever inhaler before swimming to prevent symptoms.

Swimming is a sport where fitness levels can be improved gradually and at your own pace. It is a sport that people with asthma can enjoy and in which they can have great success. This in turn can give them the confidence to participate in other sports. In 1988 Adrian Moorhouse won a gold medal at the Olympic games for swimming, proving that his asthma was no barrier to success.

As long as asthma is well controlled there is no reason why participation in sport should be restricted to swimming.

**Isn't it dangerous to use my inhaler before exercise?**

No, it is not dangerous, and in fact quite the opposite is true. Using an inhaler before exercise is quite safe, and will usually prevent asthma symptoms that are triggered during or after exercise. Two types of inhaled medicine are effective for this purpose. They are Intal (sodium cromoglicate) and the relievers such as Ventolin and Bricanyl.

Everyone with asthma should have a reliever inhaler with them at all times. Although reliever inhalers are usually used to treat and relieve symptoms of asthma they are also used to prevent *exercise-induced asthma* symptoms. Two puffs of the inhaler taken a few minutes before planned exercise is a very effective way of preventing problems.

Intal is also used as a pre-exercise treatment and is taken about half an hour before exercise. Overall in asthma, it is used much less often since the introduction of long-acting bronchodilators, which are used together with inhaled steroids (preventers) and are helpful in the treatment of exercise-induced symptoms.

Ventolin, Bricanyl and Intal are permitted for use by people with asthma participating in most competitive sports. However it is always important to check with each sporting governing body what is and what is not permitted for use. Leukotriene receptor antagonist tablets (for example, montelukast) are also helpful for exercise-induced asthma but they are used together with other asthma medicines.

### Should I stop my child playing sport?

Only under certain circumstances. It may be tempting for parents to stop their children from playing sport if this seems to bring on symptoms. If the asthma is in a bad phase and is out of control, then it is sensible to do so, because exercise may make things deteriorate further. However, the longer-term aim should be for good asthma control with **no limitations** on activities. Some of our best known athletes and sports stars have asthma and you may be hiding a potential Olympic champion!

Unfortunately there are many children who have undiagnosed or uncontrolled asthma who give the appearance of disliking sporting activities. They may feel inadequate because their sporting performance is often poor when compared with that of their school friends. We often ask children with asthma what position they play on the football pitch, and 'goalkeeper' is a frequent answer. On closer questioning we find that they may have chosen to play in goal because the position does not require too much exertion, and it therefore prevents any ridicule from their team-mates. A good test of asthma control is to ask the question again after they have received good asthma care. We have heard many times that after effective treatment they are able to play 'out' as well.

Remember that some children with asthma, on their own admission, use their asthma to get out of having to do sporting activities, even if it is not causing any problems at the time. Not all children enjoy playing sport, and in this respect children with asthma are no different from their peers.

### Are there any sports that I should avoid taking part in?

You should be able to participate in most sports despite having asthma. However, **scuba diving** is one where the situation is not always very clear. Some doctors will advise you not to dive if you have asthma, because there is a risk of dying if you have an attack when underwater. In some countries you will not be able to dive if you have asthma. We advise anyone with asthma planning a diving holiday to find out the rules in the country they are travelling to, and also at the resort that they plan to visit.

In the UK, if you have asthma, scuba diving is usually (though not always) permitted providing your asthma is well controlled (no symptoms), and that you have not needed your reliever inhaler in the 48 hours before diving. Your peak flow reading should be at your normal level at the time you want to dive. If you have asthma that is worse when the temperature is low, when you exercise or when you get stressed, you will not be able to dive. Before you dive you will need a medical certificate stating that your lung function is normal and your asthma is well controlled.

Other sports that involve the use of pressurized air or oxygen, such as **skydiving**, might require caution, but you should take specialist advice on this. For the most part, assuming your asthma is well controlled, you should be able to participate in all other sporting activities.

**I play football. Is it all right to take two more puffs at half time even though it's not 4 hours between doses?**

It is perfectly safe to take two puffs of a reliever earlier than 4 hours from the last dose. Extra puffs of inhaler at half time should be a rare occurrence, not a regular one. It is not all right to ignore the fact that, if you need this, your asthma is poorly controlled.

Regular preventive treatment should control asthma symptoms effectively. If this is not the case and you need frequent reliever treatments, as for example on the football field, then some adjustment to your regular treatment is required. Regular peak expiratory flow readings will help to identify if your asthma is well controlled. If the readings vary by more than 20% a day, from morning to evening, it is wise to consult your doctor or asthma nurse. If your asthma is better controlled, you will have more stamina on the field and your game should improve.

**I know that Becotide is a steroid – will my son be allowed to run in official sports as I thought steroids weren't allowed?**

The World Anti-Doping Agency have very strict regulations on which medicines may be used in competitive sport. Their website (see the *Appendix*) provides information and an application form for an 'Athlete's passport', which will allow your son to apply to participate and continue using his medication. The use of medicines in competitive sport is a complicated issue! The International Olympic Committee has taken steps to prevent medicine use to improve the performance of athletes, but this has led to some confusion about certain medicines that are required for medical conditions. Most asthma treatments are permitted under a therapeutic use exemption (TUE), which allows an athlete to take any medication, deemed necessary for their health, that appears on the list of prohibited substances in sport.

Athletes with asthma are also allowed to use the inhaled relievers such as Ventolin, Bricanyl, salbutamol, terbutaline, Airomir and Pulvinal [salbutamol]. The steroids used for treating asthma are in the group called corticosteroids, and are not the same as the anabolic steroids that are used illegally to improve performance and increase muscle bulk. Your son will probably be allowed to use inhaled steroids such as Becotide (beclometasone), provided he applies successfully for a TUE described above. Anyone using corticosteroid tablets or injections at the time of an event will probably be banned from competing.

Certain 'cold cures' may have substances in them that are not permitted. These include nasal decongestants containing adrenaline or isoprenaline, and any preparations with caffeine.

# *Pollution and weather*

### Are pollutants in the air causing asthma?

Surprisingly, the answer is probably not. The highest levels of asthma in the world are found in New Zealand, hardly a candidate for the world's most polluted country! Much research on the incidence of asthma around the world has shown lower levels of asthma in more polluted cities. For example, the incidence of asthma was much lower in the old Eastern German cities (that had very polluted atmospheres) than in old West Germany. Again, London in the 1950s had little asthma, but was a far more polluted city than it is now.

Nevertheless there is something about urbanization and the increasing incidence of asthma, and it cannot be good for anyone to breathe in air that is of poor quality. So the answer is that air pollution does worsen asthma, but does not explain the increases in asthma cases that we have seen in the past 50 years.

Outdoors, there are three major sources of pollutants in the air that we breathe:

- fumes from exhausts of motor vehicles that use petrol or diesel fuel

- smoke produced from burning coal, wood and gas (factories, industries and home coal fires are largely responsible for this form of pollution)

- ground-level *ozone*, which is formed by a reaction between the sun's rays and other forms of pollution such as car exhaust fumes; smoke from cigarettes, factories and fires; paint and glue fumes; and fog. Ozone is a gas, related to oxygen, which is found in small quantities in the air. This ground-level ozone is harmful to the lungs, and our pollution is producing more of it. It helps to form what is called *photochemical smog*. All of these conditions can make asthma worse. Ozone in the upper atmosphere protects us against the harmful rays of the sun. CFC propellants are contained in some asthma inhalers and contribute to the destruction of our protective ozone level. Eventually these will all be replaced by a propellant that is safer for our environment.

Indoor pollution is as important a problem as that outdoors, and is mainly due to tobacco smoke, perfumes, aerosol sprays and occasionally inefficient gas fires. There is no doubt that these substances can make asthma worse and it is worth avoiding contact with them if at all possible. The problem, of course, is that we can have little control over the air that we breathe, except for tobacco smoke in the home.

**TV weather forecasters talk about poor-quality air. Should I stay indoors or increase my treatment?**

It may be sensible to stay indoors when there is very poor air quality, but in some urban areas this might effectively put you under house arrest for long stretches of the year! Probably the most practical action you can take is to increase your preventer (inhaled steroids) treatment during these periods. If your symptoms are still uncontrolled, then you might also need to start a short course of steroid tablets – all depending on your agreed asthma action plan with your doctor or asthma nurse. Poor air quality has recently been highlighted as a cause of worsening asthma control in certain individuals. As with people whose asthma is made worse by pollen, it can be very difficult to avoid the trigger of poor air quality.

The amount and quality of information gathered about air pollution will improve greatly in the coming years, and we will all become much more aware of the day-to-day changes in our atmosphere. Information about air quality and pollen are published in the newspapers and broadcast on the radio.

### How do atmospheric conditions affect people with asthma?

Various atmospheric conditions can have an effect on asthma control. Thunderstorms seem to aggravate asthma in many people, and it has been noted that hospitals may be increasingly busy during the day or two following a thunderstorm. The most likely explanation for this is that pollen spores get released in these weather conditions.

If there is a storm, try keeping your windows closed and, if you get any asthma symptoms, increase your dose of preventer medication and start a short course of steroid tablets (if this is what you have agreed with your doctor or asthma nurse).

Research has found that people with asthma do benefit from having an agreed written asthma action plan (see Chapter 5) that is based either on best recorded peak flow or on symptoms. Reliever medication as well as steroid tablets are needed when asthma is out of control. It is a good idea to discuss the use of an action plan with your health professional.

There are important types of pollution in the atmosphere that may also make asthma worse, such as ozone (see the question above).

Weather forecasts often include mention of levels of pollen, fog and other pollution as part of their broadcast. We need to be aware of how important these forms of pollution can be and to agree how people with asthma can respond best to them. Cold dry air in winter tends to provoke asthma, while humid conditions contribute to the increase in moulds and house dust mite numbers. Although house dust mites do not qualify as 'atmospheric conditions', they are an important trigger of asthma.

**My child was admitted to hospital with a bad asthma attack after a thunderstorm. Is this common?**

There have been a few 'mini-epidemics' of acute asthma during thunderstorms. During thunderstorms, pollen grains are pulled up into the atmosphere, and explode into tiny fragments, small enough to be breathed into the lungs. Interestingly, asthma attacks following thunderstorms tend to occur in people who have hay fever, and have not previously been diagnosed with asthma. As a result, these people don't have asthma inhalers and often end up in hospital when the attacks occur. People with hay fever who suffer from wheezing episodes are prone to future asthma attacks; they should consult their doctor for a prescription for a reliever inhaler for emergency use if needed.

# Food and drink

### Can I drink alcohol when I take asthma medication?

You can certainly drink alcohol when you take asthma medication, as none of the treatments should interact with alcohol. This is not, unfortunately, the end of the story! Alcoholic drinks can sometimes be a trigger for asthma. This may be caused by the alcohol itself, or the yeast, or preservative, or by other substances derived from the grain or fruit in the drink. It is not really known whether these reactions are allergic or chemical. Allergic reactions to yeast are common, and the yeast in beer can trigger asthma in some people. Home brewing has noticeably caused an increase in yeast allergy. Quite a number of people's asthma is triggered by wine. Some cannot tolerate vintage wines but have no problem with the cheaper varieties, while others suffer the reverse. We have known people who are aware that certain alcoholic drinks affect their asthma but, rather than avoid the particular drink in question, they increase their asthma medication before imbibing! Although we can understand this approach, we cannot recommend it.

## Why do I get asthma with red wine and not white wine?

Some people get asthma from drinking both red and white wine. Others, like you, are affected only by certain types of wine, or other alcoholic drinks. Some people get asthma just from drinking soft fizzy drinks. It just goes to prove what a variable and unpredictable condition asthma is!

As a rule, red wines contain more natural chemicals than whites. There is a particular type of chemical, aldehyde, related to alcohol, which is found in red wine, and this may explain your problem. Many people find that red wine is more likely to give them hangovers, headaches or migraines, and these may also be due to this chemical.

Certain preservatives used in the manufacture of wine and soft drinks can trigger an asthma attack. The commonest of these, at least in soft drinks, is sulphur dioxide ($SO_2$). If this substance appears on the label, don't buy the product!

## I think my asthma could be due to a food allergy. I have heard about exclusion diets. What are they and should I go on one?

An exclusion diet is used in an attempt to discover whether any particular food or food additive is responsible for particular symptoms, in this case asthma symptoms. Such a diet should, in our view, be undertaken only under careful specialist medical and dietitian's supervision. This is particularly important in the case of children, who may become undernourished if their diet is not supervised by a dietitian. If you think food is making your asthma worse, you should consult your doctor or asthma nurse, who may arrange for some tests or refer you to a specialist. Young children with allergic eczema, who seem to get asthma symptoms after particular foods, should always be referred to a specialist. The main foods of concern in these children include eggs, milk and peanuts. So the first priority is to get the diagnosis correct. Then an exclusion diet may be appropriate.

There are two types of exclusion diet. In the first, any food containing a suspect ingredient, for example peanuts, egg or milk, is excluded from the diet. Peak flow measurements are made twice a day for some days before the diet is started, continued during the diet, and after normal eating is resumed. Usually the diet lasts between 10 days and 3 weeks. If peak flow measurements and symptoms become better when the food is stopped, and get worse again when including it back in your diet, the suspect food is responsible.

The second type of exclusion diet is used if no particular food is suspected, but it is felt that the asthma might be due to food allergy. In such a diet, almost everything is excluded to begin with, except for only one or two foods. Lamb and pears are usually given as examples of the basic diet allowed, because they hardly ever seem to be allergens. One by one, foods are brought back into the diet. Peak flow measurements are again recorded regularly, and within a day or so of restarting the guilty food, a fall-off in readings will be shown.

For both types of diet the whole process should be repeated twice to be absolutely sure that the changes in the asthma were not due to chance rather than the food. These diets can be difficult, time consuming and expensive. We should emphasize that it is not at all common for foodstuffs to be important triggers of asthma, and therefore expert advice should be sought before you launch into these diets.

### Are certain foods unsuitable for people with asthma?

Someone who has definite food allergy and asthma is at risk of having a life-threatening attack. However, true food allergy is not very common. This is a fairly controversial issue. Some experts believe that asthma is never, or hardly ever, related to food allergy, while others believe that it is quite common. Food allergy certainly exists and, when it is confirmed, may lead to severe asthma attacks and anaphylaxis. It is more likely to occur in people who have other allergic conditions, such as a skin allergy called urticaria, and those whose asthma is triggered by, for example, dust, pollens and animals. Therefore someone who has both food allergy (confirmed) and asthma should really be under the care of an asthma specialist.

Sometimes, asthma triggered by food allergy may take several hours to develop, and so food might not be identified as the cause. The most common food substances to cause asthma are cow's milk, nuts, peanuts, soft fruit (kiwi fruit, for example), shellfish, fish and yeast products. Food and drink additives can also cause asthma – see the answer to the next question for more details.

If you do identify a food or drink that definitely makes you wheezy, it is sensible to avoid it wherever possible. If you suffer severely, and have had anaphylactic attacks from certain foods, you should be extremely careful about checking ingredients in food you eat. It is also important to understand that it is unlikely that food will be the only trigger. Sometimes, virus infections plus exposure to foods (or other allergens) may work in combination to cause an asthma attack. So it may be difficult to pinpoint the exact cause, and regular asthma treatment may well be necessary anyway.

### Are food additives bad for people with asthma?

Some of them can be. *Tartrazine* (E numbers 102–110 and 210–219) is the most common additive causing problems for people with asthma. This is a yellow colouring that used to be found in many sweets and soft drinks, although more and more often now it is being removed. Food additives are marked on the labels of food containers in many countries, including the UK. We would advise that people with asthma should avoid tartrazine in particular. Other additives may also trigger asthma, but they may be very difficult to identify.

Sodium metabisulphate and sulphur dioxide ($SO_2$) are other examples and these are often contained in fizzy drinks.

A peak flow diary may help in finding out if a particular additive is making asthma worse. The method for using this is explained in the sections on peak expiratory flow in Chapters 3 and 5.

# Asthma and the National Health Service

Some of you may have noticed constant changes in the way that you obtain healthcare services in the community. The General Medical Services Contract in the early 1990s changed the way in which GPs worked and in particular the way they were paid. This contract introduced the concept of in-house clinics for people with chronic conditions. The latest change, the New GMS contract introduced in 2004, now requires general practices to produce evidence that they are providing a high-quality service. This determines a large proportion of their income. This includes an appointment system where the practice makes sure that patients are able to see a doctor or nurse within 48 hours. This means that there are appointments available, for both routine and emergency care, every day. Clearly patients' needs do influence the availability of appointments and, during very busy times, you might need to wait longer to be seen; however, you will always be seen on the day if it is necessary.

The other major new change is the inclusion of 10 clinical areas where the practices have to provide evidence of quality care. Two of these are respiratory – asthma and chronic obstructive pulmonary disease. In the case of asthma, the criteria include the following:

- Patients with asthma are seen once every 15 months.
- They have been offered an influenza immunization every year.
- There are records of smoking habits of their patients.

This does put a lot of additional demands on the practice and may explain why they try their best to ensure that you do attend for asthma check-ups. It is in the interest of the patient as well as the practice to make sure that this happens.

**I have to take asthma treatment regularly. Can I get any help paying for my prescriptions?**

Needing asthma treatment regularly does not mean you qualify as exempt from prescription charges. However, at present, nearly three-quarters of National Health Service patients do not pay any prescription charges. This is mainly because of their age, pregnancy or low income. If you are on Income Support you will be exempt from paying prescription charges. If you are on a low income you will need to fill in an AG1 form from the Department of Social Security and they will consider your application.

If you are not exempt from prescription charges but do need frequent prescriptions, you can apply for prepayment of your prescription charges (a *season ticket*) for a 4- or 12-month period. You will need to complete an FP95 form, available from Health Authorities, doctors' surgeries, some retail pharmacists and also the Department of Social Security. At the moment, prescription charges are such that you will be better off buying a 4-month season ticket if you are likely to need more than five prescriptions during that period, or by buying a 12-month season ticket if you are likely to need more than 16 prescriptions over the year. (The season ticket will cover all your prescriptions, not just those for your asthma treatment.) However, by the time you read this, the figures may have changed, so be careful to check that it is worth your while before paying a lump sum in advance. We have already mentioned that all asthma prescriptions are free in Wales, but not in the rest of the UK.

**I have recently been given a prescription for salbutamol. The pharmacist said it was the same medicine as the Ventolin that I am normally given, but why has it been changed?**

This is what is known as generic prescribing – a doctor prescribes a medicine by writing its generic name. Every medicine has two names – its generic name and its brand name. The generic name is the name given to each medicine when it is first developed. The brand name is the name given to the medicine when it is manufactured, and marketed, by a particular medicine company.

So, for example, salbutamol is the generic name for both Ventolin and Salbulin, which are made by different companies – these are both brand names.

Pharmaceutical companies have to obtain a licence to start manufacturing a medicine that hasn't originally been developed by them. They can then start producing it under a new and different brand name. While all the medicines can have different packaging names, there are regulations to ensure that they all have the same constituents.

The advantage of generic prescribing is almost entirely that of cost. It is usually much cheaper to provide generic medicines than brand name medicines. Perhaps, not surprisingly, the disadvantage is that the cheaper, generic medicine supplied **may** be of a lower quality. There are some safeguards to ensure the good quality of generic medicines in this country, but it is not unknown for cheap generic medicines to be imported from abroad and dispensed. In the UK about half of all medicines are prescribed generically. In asthma the proportion is lower than this, probably because doctors and those with asthma like to be sure of the quality, the colour and feel of the inhaler devices that are being prescribed.

**My doctor says he feels my treatment is too expensive. What will happen?**

We all have to be cost conscious these days, and there is no doubt that asthma is expensive for everyone. A conservative estimate puts the cost of asthma to the country at around £889 million per year, in terms of National Health Service costs and social security payments. Lost productivity at work costs a further £1.2 billion.

A large proportion of the cost of treating asthma is due to hospital attendance and admissions. Correct treatment, even though it may seem expensive, costs less and is more effective (both for the individual's health and for NHS finances) than poor asthma control. It costs about £65 for 1 year's treatment, in primary care, for mild asthma at standard doses of beclometasone and salbutamol. The medicine costs for more severe asthma could reach £1000 per year.

In our view, GPs should be encouraged to resist pressure to cut prescribing costs for asthma just for the sake of it. Instead they should concentrate on choosing whatever treatment is best for the individual patient. Good asthma management, including preventive treatment, not only makes people better and able to live normal lives, but can also cut NHS costs by reducing hospital admissions, as well as reducing the number of days lost from work or school.

Those are our views but, if your GP genuinely feels that your treatment is too expensive, you will need to discuss this carefully with him or her, and perhaps the Primary Care Organization. Your local Patient Forum represents your interests as a consumer of health care, and they may also be able to give you advice.

## *The long-term outlook*

**Does a good control of symptoms make the long-term outlook better for me?**

Good control of asthma reduces symptoms, making a person feel better. Very often people are unaware of how much they are tolerating asthma symptoms and, if effective treatment removes these, they then suddenly feel dramatically better. Thus there is no doubt that 'quality of life' is improved by a good control of symptoms. There is also good evidence that an effective control of asthma symptoms reduces the number of acute attacks. These benefits are to do with the short-term outcome of asthma, and what happens in the next few years. We cannot say for sure yet that the outcome in 15, 20 or 30 years will be improved by good asthma control. We believe that it will be, but the research studies to prove or disprove it will take many years to complete.

In the meantime, we feel sure that the short- and medium-term benefits of good asthma control are sufficient to justify regular treatment, as long as it is effective.

**As I get older, will my asthma get worse?**

This depends on how old you are when you ask this question! It used to be thought that nearly all children 'grew out of' their asthma by the end of their teens. Research has now shown that the outlook is not quite so good. Only about one in three lose their asthma completely. A further third either have a great reduction in symptoms, or their asthma stops only temporarily. The other third continue to suffer from asthma, although often in a milder form. In adults, the longer the asthma has been present, the more likely it is to have caused some permanent damage to the airways. In general, asthma does get worse as a person gets older, although even in adults asthma can improve or even disappear for many years.

There are other factors involved in getting older that may make asthma seem worse. Lung function decreases with age in everybody, so that we have less in reserve when we require extra air. Other conditions such as chronic bronchitis and emphysema also become more common with increasing age, increasing the problems posed by asthma. (See the section on **Related conditions** in Chapter 2 for more information about bronchitis and emphysema.) The best way to prevent asthma becoming worse with age is to:

- avoid smoking
- treat acute episodes early
- take preventive treatment regularly
- maintain general health and fitness as much as possible.

### Can adult asthma, like childhood asthma, be grown out of?

As we keep saying in this book, asthma is a very variable condition. It is certainly possible for asthma to disappear in adults, just as it does in children. However, you are far less likely to 'grow out' of adult asthma. People with late-onset asthma tend to have continuous symptoms. It will certainly vary in severity from time to time and maybe from season to season. Other than upper respiratory tract infections (such as the common cold) it is not easy to identify obvious triggers.

Sometimes late-onset asthma can start because the patient has been prescribed a medicine for another medical condition. Examples of this are aspirin, some of the anti-arthritis medicines (NSAIDs) and beta-blockers (see the **Glossary** for more details about these groups of medicines). Even eye drops that are prescribed for glaucoma can contain beta-blocker medicines and make asthma worse. If it seems likely that any of these medicines are triggering asthma symptoms, in some cases stopping the medicine can lead to a full recovery. Talk to your doctor or asthma nurse about this, especially if the medicines have been prescribed by them, so that alternatives can be prescribed. In these few cases, one could perhaps say the asthma has been 'cured'. Similarly, people who develop occupational asthma often improve when they are no longer exposed to the occupational trigger factor.

### Could my asthma be affecting my heart?

If your asthma is well controlled, you have no need to worry. People sometimes get palpitations after taking reliever treatment and worry that their heart is being damaged. This is not the case.

Some people get chest tightness when their asthma is not well controlled or if they have been exposed to an asthma trigger such as exercise. This tightness can be around the breast bone or feel as though the chest is being squeezed as if in a vice. If your reliever inhaler makes this tightness and discomfort go away you can be fairly confident that it is due to your asthma and not your heart. Heart pains (angina) can be referred down the arm and shoulder. Talk to your doctor or asthma nurse about your concerns. They may feel it worthwhile for you to have a heart-reading test (an electrocardiogram, or ECG) to make sure that you do not have a heart problem.

Uncontrolled asthma and severe asthma attacks may reduce the amount of oxygen that can be breathed into the lungs, and then transported in the bloodstream. This shortage of oxygen may put a strain on the heart, particularly if it is severe or if it continues for many hours or days. If there is a shortage of oxygen in the blood, the heart tries to overcome this by pumping faster and harder, and the heart may get exhausted as a result of this extra work. In addition the heart muscle itself may suffer as a result of a shortage of oxygen. In practical terms this is rarely a problem, except in very severe attacks, or if the heart has already been weakened from some other problem. Still, it emphasizes that it is very important to avoid severe attacks, and to try to maintain the best possible control of asthma for the rest of the time.

Regular exercise helps to keep the circulation in good condition. This enables the heart to increase its work when the person has an asthma attack. Smoking and other air pollutants interfere with the body's ability to carry oxygen in the bloodstream, and this puts further strain on the heart.

### Will I need to be on oxygen when I get older?

This is very unlikely unless you have other severe chest problems such as chronic bronchitis or emphysema (see the section on *Related conditions* in Chapter 2 for more information about these). For such people, their lung function tends to become worse and worse as the years go by, and having asthma as well may leave them very short of oxygen all of the time. Under these conditions oxygen in the home (domiciliary oxygen) may be needed. This is provided under the care of a hospital specialist in chest diseases. Modern equipment can extract oxygen from the air and concentrate it so there is no need to have great big oxygen cylinders cluttering up the front room. The oxygen can be breathed through a small cannula (a soft plastic pipe) which fits neatly into the nose passages. This is much more comfortable than the old style of having a large mask clamped over the face for many hours a day. Sometimes, during severe asthma attacks, high doses of oxygen will be needed for a short time, but only to relieve the symptoms of the attack more rapidly.

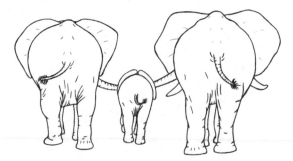

**Personal action plan – things you might wish to discuss
with your doctor or asthma nurse**

If you want to adjust your asthma medicines, you will need a
personal action plan (self-management plan) from your doctor or
asthma nurse.

- If you have developed asthma for the first time as an adult –
  check the Health and Safety Executive and Asthma UK
  websites (see *Appendix*) and see if your occupation is linked
  with asthma. If so, discuss this with your doctor or asthma
  nurse; you might need to do a 2–4 hourly peak flow chart and
  you may need referral to a specialist in occupational medicine.

- If you are due to travel, make sure you that have an action
  plan, spare asthma medicines and information on the health
  services at your destination in case your asthma is
  troublesome.

- If you think food may be triggering your asthma, discuss this.
  You might need food allergy tests and you might need an
  adrenaline injection to carry round with you. In addition it
  would be worth considering registering with MedicAlert (see
  *Appendix*) who would add you to their database list of
  people with important medical conditions. There is an initial
  charge and you can obtain a necklace, bracelet (or dog tag
  or Velcro wrist band) engraved with information about your
  allergies as well as contact details on accessing your medical
  details from MedicAlert. There is a small yearly charge to
  keep your details on the database and these should be
  updated as necessary. This information can be very useful
  and in some situations life saving, where immediate
  information may be needed about your allergies.

# 7
# Children and asthma

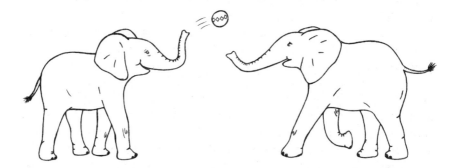

In this chapter you will learn about:

- asthma in infants and childhood

- useful tips to help you give asthma inhalers to infants and toddlers

- asthma at school and the use of inhalers to promote independence

- potential side effects of asthma medicines and their safety

- asthma triggers

- the benefits of exercise

- asthma in adolescents.

224

Asthma is the most common chronic medical condition affecting children in the UK. We know that the number of children in the population who suffer from asthma is increasing. In an average primary school class in the UK there will be three or more children who have asthma and are receiving treatment for the condition.

Education authorities have established policies to address the issue of children with asthma and other long-term conditions in schools. In some areas of the country, school nurses with asthma training are helping teachers to learn more about asthma and to enable children with asthma to cope with their condition when at school.

Until recently, children with asthma were not always diagnosed with the condition or treated. They were just thought to be 'chesty' or to have repeated episodes of bronchitis. Now we appreciate how common asthma in childhood is, we can be more confident about making the diagnosis. If asthma is not diagnosed and treated, many children will suffer unnecessarily from respiratory symptoms. This means that they may have time off school and miss out on many social activities, both at home and at school. The days when children with asthma are regarded as delicate and highly strung should be long gone. Many of the questions in this chapter aim to provide reassurance that it is possible for them to have a normal lifestyle.

In this chapter we discuss asthma across the spectrum of childhood; from infancy to adolescence. Asthma in infancy is often difficult to diagnose and treat, and presents a number of issues for children, parents and health professionals alike. Asthma in early childhood varies widely, from occasional symptoms that occur only with coughs and colds (viral infections) to more persistent and troublesome symptoms, often related to allergic triggers. Many children do seem to 'grow out' of their asthma as they get older, especially if it is triggered only by viral infections.

In early childhood, asthma is more common in boys than in girls and usually improves with increasing age. In girls, asthma can be troublesome as they get older and symptoms are usually more persistent. In addition, asthma is more likely to occur for the first time in the teenage years in girls than in boys. Adolescent children report more symptoms than we were previously aware of and only around one in three lose their asthma completely.

# How and when does asthma start?

### How young can asthma be diagnosed?

Asthma can be diagnosed in children under 1 year old but it is essential that other more serious diseases are considered and not missed. Any child who has frequent respiratory symptoms in the first year of life, such as wheezing or coughing that persists for weeks, should be referred to a specialist in childhood chest problems to find the cause of the problems.

If a detailed medical history is taken, it will usually be sufficient to confirm the diagnosis of asthma. This medical history needs to take account of the chest problems taking note of:

- when they first appeared
- what sets them off
- how frequently they appear
- whether they get better after any particular treatment.

However, the diagnosis is often difficult to confirm as the required special tests can be done only in specialist children's facilities.

In very young children there are some clues to the diagnosis of asthma. These are children who:

- cough a lot, especially at night
- wheeze from time to time, especially with colds
- get colds that go to the chest and take several weeks to get better
- have persistent symptoms of cough and wheeze even when they do not have colds
- cough, wheeze or get chest tightness when they get excited or run around
- get better after anti-asthma treatment.

In addition a family history of asthma or other allergic diseases such as eczema or hay fever makes the diagnosis of asthma more likely in a child who gets lots of chest symptoms. Children living in a house with a smoker are also more likely to develop asthma.

**The doctor thinks my baby son has asthma. Why can't they do any tests so they can tell me definitely what the problem is?**

As we have already said in the previous question, there are no tests to confirm the diagnosis of asthma in babies and very young children, except in specialist children's hospitals. These tests may be used only in research projects.

Peak flow tests (see the sections on peak expiratory flow in Chapters 3 and 5) can be used at a later stage to confirm the diagnosis of asthma but this may not be until your child is 5 or 6 years of age or older. These involve taking some readings using a peak flow meter or by more specialized blowing tests using equipment called a spirometer. Spirometers are beginning to be used more often by doctors and asthma nurses in general practice, but it can be difficult to obtain good test results in younger children, unless the doctors or nurses are really experienced in carrying them out in children. In your baby's situation these tests are not possible.

For your baby son, the diagnosis of asthma will be made after the doctor has examined him and asked you lots of questions. You will also be asked about your own health and other members of the family, because a family history of asthma makes the diagnosis of asthma more likely for your son. Putting all this information together will help the doctor come to a decision as to the likelihood of an asthma diagnosis. It is really frustrating for you if the doctor says he thinks your baby son has asthma, because you want to know definitely, but this is not always possible. If the doctor thinks that your son has asthma, your son is likely to be prescribed anti-asthma medicines to see if they help. Clearly if they do help, it is good news, but it will also help confirm the diagnosis of asthma.

**Our child has asthma – whose fault is it? There is no history of it in our family.**

Without knowing the precise circumstances we cannot be sure, but it would be wrong to 'blame' somebody for the development of asthma in your child.

Many children with asthma have a family history of asthma, eczema or allergy (e.g. house dust mite allergy or hay fever). These children inherit the asthma tendency in their genes. The asthma may show itself only when the child comes into contact with the relevant trigger factor such as dust, cats, exercise or a cold. Some children develop asthma even though no one else in the immediate family has it, but there is usually some asthma, hay fever or eczema on one or other side of the family.

There is a connection between smoking and respiratory symptoms in children. A child who is exposed to cigarette smoke in early life (while in the uterus and during the first few years after birth) is at greater risk of developing asthma. This is especially so if the mother has asthma, but can also happen to children where there is no family history. It is desirable and sensible for anyone who smokes and is thinking of becoming pregnant to stop smoking first. Reducing exposure to cigarette smoke is sensible advice and adopting a non-smoking policy in the home is ideal, but not always possible.

**My dad lives with us and smokes. I'm worried about my daughter because she is always coughing. I'm sure the smoke is making her worse. How can I get him to stop smoking?**

Smoking is known to increase respiratory illnesses in children and, if there is asthma as well, is a recognized trigger of asthma symptoms. The issue of smoking is a sensitive one, but do talk to your dad about your concerns. We are sure he doesn't want his grandchild to be troubled by his smoking, but it is a very addictive habit and is very difficult to stop. He may want to stop smoking but not know how or what help is available. Wanting to stop is the first stage of quitting smoking. Why don't you suggest he talks to his doctor, practice nurse or local pharmacist about what help is available. There are many very effective smoking cessation support programmes in place in the National Health Service (NHS), which may help your dad. Nicotine replacement treatment is available on prescription; anyone enrolled on the National Health Service 'STOP' smoking programme is eligible for cheaper nicotine patches.

If he does not want to stop smoking, ask him either to smoke outside or at least not in the same room as your daughter and the rest of the family. The problem is that the smoke clings to clothing and your child will still be affected by the smell of the smoke particles when dad comes into the house. There are, of course, health and financial benefits to stopping smoking for your father, but he probably knows that. Try to be supportive and encouraging if he attempts to stop smoking and is unsuccessful. Many people do not succeed at their first attempt. It's always worth trying again.

### Is asthma more common in boys or girls?

Childhood asthma is undoubtedly more common in boys. In the UK it is somewhere between two and three times more common in boys, although some surveys have suggested an even higher ratio. Asthma is also more common in boys in most parts of the world. The reasons for the difference are not clear and there does not seem to be any difference in the nature or severity of asthma.

Studies do not suggest that the difference between boys and girls is because of their different genetic make up. There may be other factors earlier in childhood. For example, we know that boys have smaller airways as babies, and are more prone to respiratory infections than girls. In adult life, men and women are affected in more or less equal numbers; however, in the age range 20–40 years, women seem to be affected more than men. There is also some evidence that late-onset asthma is more common in women. Boys are more likely than girls to 'lose' their asthma in adolescence. This also helps to explain how the ratios come to be more equal in adults.

**My son is 7 years old. How can I find out how severe his asthma is?**

The amount of treatment your son needs to control his asthma will give an indication as to how severe it is. Not everyone fits neatly into a category of mild, moderate or severe asthma especially if their asthma is well controlled. It isn't always easy for you to judge the severity of your son's asthma, although we are sure you will have some idea. It is more difficult if you have not had experience of seeing other people with asthma. Another problem is that even people with mild occasional asthma symptoms can sometimes develop bad asthma quite quickly. Only a few of the very high numbers of children with asthma have to be admitted to hospital because of an attack, so, if your son has needed to go into hospital, that puts him towards the moderate to severe end of the range.

Make an appointment with your doctor or asthma nurse and they will be able to make an assessment as to how severe your son's asthma is, at the moment. This is done not only by carrying out blowing tests of peak flow (PEF), but also by asking you carefully about your son's symptoms now and in the past. Asthma is such a changeable condition that it is important to keep a check on all these things. It may be an idea for your son to use a peak flow meter for the few weeks before he attends the practice for an asthma check-up. Ongoing use of a PEF test can also help you to assess your son's condition more accurately and to check the severity of any episode of asthma. (See the sections on peak expiratory flow in Chapters 3 and 5, and Chapter 8 on *Emergencies*.)

**My son is 5 years old and has asthma. Is there any connection with the immunizations he has had?**

**No!** There is no connection between routine childhood immunizations and asthma. Routine childhood immunizations protect against potentially life-threatening disease and they do not cause or trigger asthma. Any chesty episode that occurs around the time of immunization is purely coincidental.

# *Infants*

**When my 6-month-old daughter coughs a lot, should I give her cough mixture as well as her inhalers?**

Coughing is a common symptom of asthma and, although it is tempting to use cough medicines, there is no evidence that they help. Many health professionals believe that cough mixtures are a waste of money; you would be well advised to look at the British National Formulary entries for these medicines (see *Appendix*). Using cough mixtures can create a false sense of security because you may think no other treatment is needed. There are also possible dangerous side effects from taking cough medicines, particularly if they contain codeine, which can have a harmful effect on breathing. Cough mixtures containing codeine or similar compounds should be avoided in children and should **not** be given to children under 1 year of age. It is best to use the asthma medicines as advised by the doctor or asthma nurse, and to seek help if they don't work.

One of the main problems in an infant of this age is actually getting the asthma medicines into the lungs. Young children often do not tolerate a face mask and inhaler device very well, and it requires a lot of patience to get them to accept them. Once the device is tolerated the medicines have a better chance of working and the symptoms will often disappear.

**Are those children who suffer from croup in infancy more at risk of developing asthma?**

No. Croup causes narrowing of the larynx (voice box) and upper part of the trachea (windpipe) and, in this age group, is caused by respiratory virus infections (e.g. the common cold). Croup results in a painful, barking cough and difficulty in breathing for infants and younger children. It often affects the same child on a number of occasions, but it is a separate condition from asthma, and does not put the child at any increased risk of developing asthma. There is another condition that infants get, called *bronchiolitis,* and this does have a link with asthma later in childhood.

### Do I hold my baby down if she is fighting the facemask of her spacer device?

We believe you should never hold your child down to give her the asthma medicines. It can be really difficult to get young children to accept a face mask and spacer and it requires a lot of patience on your behalf especially if she is chesty and you are worried. Although we normally say there must be a good seal between the mask and around the nose and mouth, if your daughter is very wheezy or breathless and is fighting the face mask, try holding the face mask a little distance away from her face. This is sometimes enough for a little of the medicine to be sucked in as she breathes, giving some relief. Once the airways start to open, babies often start to relax more, and will accept the mask more readily.

When your daughter is well, try to get her used to the spacer device and mask. Make it as much fun as you can, and very much a game. If she refuses the device or starts to get upset, put it away and try again later. Gradually your daughter will come to accept the device but it will take time and patience. If you get upset, so will your daughter. Sometimes involving other people to give her the inhaler device, such as nursery staff, can be helpful. Giving her the asthma inhalers when she is not too tired and irritable may also be helpful.

There are several different types of face masks and spacer devices and some may be accepted more readily than others. Sometimes smaller devices with a face mask or one that is brightly coloured are more acceptable than the larger spacers, but this is not always the case. Don't be tempted to give her the inhaler device when she is asleep. If she wakes up with a mask over her face this may upset and frighten her.

### Will giving inhalers to a baby prevent asthma developing?

It is not possible to tell which babies will develop asthma in the future, and there is no justification for giving anti-asthma treatment before the condition has developed. At present the main reason for prescribing inhaled asthma treatment is to control and reduce respiratory symptoms owing to asthma. Another reason is as a 'therapeutic test', i.e. to see if the child gets better with asthma treatment; this frequently helps in making the diagnosis. Good symptom control in the early stages of asthma means fewer problems in later life. Early treatment of asthma will reduce the risks of any long-term problems and may also shorten the duration of asthma symptoms.

**My 10-month-old baby recently saw a specialist because he gets very wheezy when he has a cold. The specialist mentioned viral wheezing one minute and then baby and infant asthma. I'm confused. What does he mean?**

These terms are confusing, but they are all used to describe wheezing illnesses in young children. Virus infections are the most common trigger of asthma and in young children they trigger wheezing and other respiratory symptoms such as coughing. At 10 months it is sometimes very difficult to say for sure whether your baby has asthma as there are no easily available tests to confirm the diagnosis, so these terms are used. Your specialist will have asked you lots of questions such as when the wheezing started, what sets it off, family history of asthma, hay fever, whether anyone smokes in the family and so on. The specialist will piece this information together to decide what the problem is most likely to be, because he will want to make sure that the wheezing is not a result of other conditions.

The specialist has used the terms viral wheezing, baby asthma and infant asthma so is apparently happy that there is nothing more serious going on, which is good news. The specialist may recommend a trial of asthma inhaler treatments to see if they help relieve the wheezing symptoms. At your baby's age they are not always effective, because getting the asthma medicines in can be quite difficult, even if a spacer device and face mask are used. Inhalers are preferred to asthma syrup medicines because smaller doses of medicine can be given, but asthma syrup is still prescribed sometimes.

The other good news is that children who get wheezy in early childhood as a result of viral infections, but who have no family history of asthma (or other associated conditions), do seem to grow out of the symptoms as they get older.

# *Childhood*

### Does vomiting set off attacks of asthma in children?

Vomiting does not set off an asthma attack in children; it is more likely to be the result of the asthma. Vomiting is quite common in young children with asthma who are troubled by frequent coughing. Frequent coughing especially at night is a sign that the asthma is not under control. In young children mucus from sore (inflamed) airways is usually swallowed because they do not like spitting it out. Pressure from distended lungs and coughing may push down on the diaphragm, and squeeze the stomach, leading to vomiting. The vomit contains lots of mucus (slimy phlegm). Children usually feel much better after they have vomited, probably because there is less pressure on the diaphragm. If a child's asthma is not under control and they are coughing and vomiting, additional asthma treatment is usually needed.

### Is it safe to let my 8-year-old decide how much Ventolin to take when she is away from me?

Yes it is, but it will depend on your child, her understanding and her physical capabilities: 8-year-old children can be very good at managing their own asthma, and can often stick to simple instructions. Most will be able to understand that they should take their Ventolin (salbutamol) if they get asthma symptoms, as well as taking it before exercise, in order to stop exercise-induced symptoms. For these children it seems perfectly reasonable that they should be allowed to decide when to take the Ventolin. A report from Asthma UK (previously known as the National Asthma Campaign) found that most children over the age of 7 were quite capable of deciding when they needed their inhaler.

Perhaps the first and most important thing to remember is that, even if a child takes more than their usual dose of Ventolin inhaler, it will not do them any harm apart from increasing their pulse rate for a short time, and making them feel rather trembly.

If your daughter is using more and more Ventolin than usual and it doesn't seem to make any difference to her asthma symptoms, this is a sign that her asthma is getting worse. Your daughter needs to know that, if there are problems, she must get help from a grown-up or ask one of her friends to go and fetch help. You will need to make sure your daughter knows:

- what her Ventolin (or other) reliever inhaler does

- when she should take it

- how much Ventolin she takes each time

- what to do if it doesn't work

- when she can repeat the dose

- what to do if it still doesn't work and how to get help.

Make sure your daughter's school have this information written down and also who to contact in an emergency. If there is any doubt, they should dial 999 for emergency help.

One of the main problems for children occurs if they are using an inhaler device that they cannot use very well on their own. Metered dose inhalers (spray inhalers) are difficult to use for people of all ages. In children under the age of about 12 years of age they should not be used unless they are used with a spacer device. This is because of the difficulties of coordinating both pressing the inhaler and breathing in at the same time.

A dry powder or a breath-activated device is easier for your daughter to use when she is away from home, but these too can be difficult to use if asthma symptoms are severe. A device which makes it easy to check how much Ventolin (or salbutamol) is used is best. These devices can help you monitor how much medicine has been taken and how much is left in the device. The Diskhaler using Ventodisks has eight single doses of Ventolin in each disk. The Ventolin Accuhaler is a multidose device with a numerical counter and contains 60 doses.

Alternatively there are other dry powder devices containing salbutamol (which is the same active ingredient as Ventolin). This widens the choice of inhaler device options to include devices such as the salbutamol Pulvinal, the salbutamol Easyhaler, or the salbutamol Clickhaler. The Pulvinal has a transparent inhaler body so your daughter can see how much medicine is left while the Clickhaler has a numbered counter containing 200 doses.

The Easi-Breathe device is a metered dose inhaler but, once the lid has been opened, the asthma medicine is not released until you breathe in. This avoids the problems of coordination and many children of 8 years of age can use this device really well. Additionally there is the Airomir Autohaler device, which is similar, but you need to lift a lever on the top of the device before breathing in the medicine from the inhaler. When you breathe in, the medicine is released.

### Could asthma cause my child not to grow properly, because his asthma is always troublesome?

Uncontrolled asthma can certainly be responsible for poor growth in children. Children with bad asthma often have delayed puberty. This means that they are often shorter than their friends in their early teens, but then 'catch up' in their late teens.

Growth hormone, which stimulates growth in the young body, is normally released in bursts during sleep and also during vigorous exercise. If your child does not sleep well or is unable to play sports because of poor asthma control, then less of his growth hormone will be released. Children with severe asthma also tend be underweight because they have much higher energy requirements than normal.

Your child may need reassurance that he will grow in height. He may be quite sensitive about his lack of height in comparison with some of his friends. There is a wide variety in what is 'normal' and reassurance may be all that is required. Make sure you talk to your child about any concerns he may have and ask that his height is checked at least 6 monthly, or whenever you attend for an asthma review. If his height is plotted on a special growth chart, you and your son can check what progress there is. If you still have concerns about his lack of height, do talk to your doctor or asthma nurse and they may refer you to a growth specialist for advice.

**Is there any chance that I might give my child an overdose of her asthma treatment?**

Asthma medicines are safe if they are given at the recommended doses and overdoses are unlikely.

High doses of the reliever medicines (such as Ventolin – salbutamol; Bricanyl – terbutaline) are life-saving in acute asthma situations. Giving 25 puffs or doses from a salbutamol inhaler is equal to a 2.5 mg dose from a nebulizer, a dose commonly used in young children. Side effects of high doses are a fast heart rate and trembling but these effects are not long lasting. Sometimes it is not recognized that urgent medical help is needed despite the high doses of reliever medicines needed. This is a potentially serious problem. Additional medicines, such as a short course of prednisolone tablets or inhaled steroids, will be needed to gain control of asthma symptoms. Always seek help if your child's asthma fails to get better after the usual treatment.

Inhaled steroids (preventers) have a recommended upper dose limit. Your doctor or asthma nurse will plan with you the dose that your child should take. They will refer to the British Asthma Guideline, which suggests the best starting doses of inhaled steroids and when to add in other medicines. These guidelines specify doses that should be used across different age groups.

Leukotriene receptor antagonists, e.g. Singulair or montelukast, are chewable tablets. Side effects are usually minimal but they may occasionally cause tummy aches or headaches.

There are no known risks of overdose with Intal (sodium cromoglicate) or Tilade (nedocromil). However, people with asthma who take these medications without inhaled steroids, may suffer from more asthma attacks because they are not as good at preventing attacks.

It is possible to overdose people with the theophylline group of medicines such as aminophylline, Nuelin (theophylline) or Slo-Phyllin (theophylline). Fortunately, these are not used as often now because other asthma medicines are available, which are usually very effective. If theophylline medicines are used, they should always be used with caution and it may be necessary to have occasional blood tests to make sure that the blood levels are not too high.

In summary, asthma treatments are safe and effective when used at the correct dose to control symptoms. Asthma medicines should be reviewed at each asthma check with your doctor or asthma nurse.

### How old does a child have to be before he can be skin prick tested for allergies?

Skin prick tests can be carried out at any age, even on a newborn baby. They are painless when carried out by an experienced person. A negative test on the skin does not prove that a child does not react internally to an allergen. A positive test is a bit more helpful, in that it does confirm the presence of the allergic tendency (atopy) but it does not confirm the diagnosis of asthma. In a young child, the medical history is usually sufficient to confirm the diagnosis of asthma. When the child is older, special blowing test results will add to the overall picture and diagnosis of asthma. If a child has asthma, skin tests will not affect the treatment decisions.

Skin tests may be helpful if you want to check if you are allergic to, for example, cats. A positive cat allergy skin test may help you make the decision against cat ownership. (See Chapter 4 for a question on this.)

### My child has asthma – how can I help make her lungs stronger?

Although it may seem surprising, your daughter's lungs are not necessarily any weaker than those of a child who does not have asthma. If asthma is controlled by giving the correct asthma medicines, which reduce the inflammation in the airways, the lungs will function absolutely normally. The best way for you to help your daughter is for you to encourage her to lead a full and active life with as few restrictions as possible. In this respect physical exercise is very important. Swimming is definitely one of the best activities to encourage physical development, and this is an ideal activity for a child with asthma.

In those few children with very severe asthma, special breathing exercises, taught by physiotherapists, may be necessary to improve the function of the lungs. Talk to your doctor or asthma nurse if your daughter is in this group.

**Can a child with asthma be underweight?**

Children with severe or poorly controlled asthma are quite often underweight. If there is a long delay in diagnosing asthma, children may be underweight and then improve considerably once treatment is started.

Research has been carried out into the calorie intake needed for growth in children with asthma. It has been shown that they have greater energy (calorie) needs than children of the same age and weight who do not have asthma. This must be something to do with the extra effort required for day-to-day living with uncontrolled asthma. During acute asthma attacks, children may use up vast amounts of energy and, unless they make up for it quite quickly afterwards by eating well, they will lose weight.

Once the asthma is well controlled with the right treatment, the child can catch up rapidly in terms of weight and growth. We have all seen children who are underweight with poorly controlled asthma who have improved dramatically, once their asthma comes under control.

In a similar way, poorly controlled asthma may result in a child failing to gain height, as well as weight. Although there are concerns that high doses of steroid treatment may affect growth, it is more often the asthma that affects growth rather than the treatment. Make sure that your doctor or asthma nurse checks your child's height and weight at the asthma review. This can be recorded and any changes followed closely.

# At school

### Should I tell a teacher that I have asthma?

Yes. It is important for your teachers to know about any health issues that may interfere with your schooling. For example, in your science classes you may be working with substances that make your asthma worse. If your teachers know about this, they may be able to modify the experiments you are doing – perhaps letting you use a fume cupboard so that you do not risk inhaling anything that could cause your asthma to get worse.

If pupils can let their teachers know how their asthma affects them, it may be possible to prevent future problems. PE and other sporting activities are the most important area of school life where the teacher needs to be well informed about asthma, and sensitive to the pupil's health needs. Unfortunately, our experience is that this is often not the case. Amongst children of all ages, problems with activities at school are quite common.

Asthma UK, which is a charity for people with asthma (see *Appendix*), has done a great deal to improve the knowledge and management of asthma in schools. They have produced school packs, and also a school asthma card, which is completed by the doctor or asthma nurse. This then provides very helpful information for the teacher as to what asthma treatment the child is taking, as well as what they should do if the child has worsening asthma or a severe asthma attack. Asthma UK's website has useful information about all aspects of asthma.

### My teachers don't like me to use my inhalers at school. Is it all right to miss my lunchtime dose?

It is always best to take your asthma treatment as prescribed by your doctor or asthma nurse, but we are not sure what you mean by your lunchtime dose! Nowadays preventer asthma medicines are taken twice or even once a day. If you are taking your preventer asthma inhalers more often, you should ask your GP practice or hospital clinic about your treatment.

The only asthma inhaler that you need to carry around with you is your blue reliever inhaler. Usually this is taken 'as needed' but, if your asthma has been troublesome or you have a cold, then you may need to use it more often. If you are breathless, wheezy, coughing a lot or have chest tightness, you must use your blue reliever inhaler. You may also need to use your reliever inhaler before any sporting activities to prevent exercise symptoms. If you are using more of your blue inhaler than normal or it is not working as well as it usually does, you do need to get your asthma checked by your doctor or asthma nurse.

Unfortunately, some teachers do not realize the importance of taking reliever asthma treatment when it is needed. They may say that they find it disruptive to school routine if children need to use them. This is probably because their schools have a policy that requires all medicines including asthma inhalers to be locked away for safety purposes. For asthma, it would be far less disruptive if you and others with asthma had access to their inhalers at all times or were allowed to keep the inhaler with them. An inhaler is of no benefit if it is locked away and you are on a sports field or playground.

Perhaps you and your parents could speak to the school about the problems you are having. Alternatively, your GP practice could ask the school nurse to discuss the issue of access to inhalers with the teachers at your school. Other possibilities are for your GP practice to write to the school about the problems, or make contact with the parent governors for the school. Sometimes the main problem is that people just don't know about asthma. You could suggest that the teacher has a look at Asthma UK's website for information about asthma.

### Can my son keep his inhaler with him in school?

As we have said in the answer to the previous question, some schools have policies on whether or not children are allowed to keep their inhalers on them during school time. Unfortunately, too many of them have strict policies about all medicines being locked away, so that asthma treatments are inaccessible. Even if your son is not allowed to keep his inhaler in his pocket, he should have free access to it at all times. Delay in taking reliever treatment can lead to a severe attack. Where possible, schools should involve the parents as to whether or not the inhalers are held by the pupil or by the school. For younger children, it seems sensible that the inhalers should be kept by the teacher in the classroom. For some older children at primary school, and for all those at secondary schools, the inhalers should be kept by the children themselves.

**Why won't teachers give my daughter her inhaler?**

This is quite a common problem. One of the difficulties for teachers is that the conditions of their employment do not include giving medicines or supervising a pupil to take them. However, our experience is that many are happy to supervise inhaler use but not make the decision to give it. Anyone taking on the responsibility of administering medicines should always have appropriate training and guidance.

In an emergency situation (for example an unexpected acute asthma attack – see Chapter 8), school staff are required to act as any reasonable or prudent parent would. This may include administering medication. For more information on the legal aspects of managing pupils with medical needs, have a look at the Department of Health's *Managing medicines in schools and early years settings* (see *Appendix*).

**How can I convince other people (e.g. teachers) of the seriousness of my child's condition?**

If possible, try to arrange a time when you can talk with your child's teacher without being disturbed. Unless you are absolutely sure of your facts, we suggest that you take some reading material on the subject of asthma with you; you can then leave this behind for the teacher to read. You could also take this opportunity to explain about the asthma medicines that your child is taking, and the importance of making sure that they are readily available when your child is at school. You may find it more convenient to get a reliever inhaler for your child to be kept especially for use at school.

It may be worth talking to the school nurse about any problems your child is having at school. If you are not sure who your school nurse is, your GP practice will be able to help you. Asthma UK produces an excellent schools information pack (see *Appendix* for their address, and also see the answer to the next question). Their website is worth visiting for further information.

### Will teachers understand my son's asthma?

All the surveys carried out to date show that school teachers have only a very limited understanding of asthma and its management. Very few teachers have received any teaching or training about the condition. A survey, testing the knowledge of school teachers in eight schools in London in 1990, looked at this. It revealed that, while most teachers realized that asthma could be influenced by emotional factors, only one in three knew that taking asthma treatment before games could prevent asthma attacks. We believe that all the good work done to raise awareness of asthma in schools by Asthma UK has helped the situation, but we know there are still some problems.

Most of the teachers in the survey knew very little indeed about the various treatments, and unfortunately nearly half of them said that they would not allow children with asthma to keep their inhalers with them. Some felt that children might overdose themselves, while others believed that children should be 'protected' from inhalers in case they developed an 'unhealthy attachment' to them! It seems that the chief problem is that teachers have felt poorly informed and ill-equipped to cope with children who have asthma. This has often been seen by parents as a lack of interest by the teacher.

Asthma UK (see *Appendix* for their address) has produced a *Schools Asthma Policy Document* to help improve asthma management at school. Schools can adapt this document to meet the needs of their school. The document puts special emphasis on the importance of preventing asthma symptoms – particularly in relation to sporting activities – and the necessity of providing easy access for the children to their inhalers at all times. It also gives guidance on what to do if a child has an asthma attack.

We feel that teachers are becoming far better informed about asthma. It will not be until all the teachers' colleges include training sessions on asthma, and all school teachers receive in-service training on the subject, that the situation will improve.

**What if another child at school gets hold of my daughter's inhaler and uses it?**

This is a common worry for both parents and teachers because they fear that these medicines may be dangerous if given to the wrong person. We can assure you, however, that no harm will come to any child who used your daughter's inhaler – whatever treatment she takes. Unfortunately, some children do sometimes use or play with metered dose inhalers that belong to children with asthma by spraying them around. This wastes the medicine and the real concern is that there won't be enough asthma inhaler medicine when your child really needs it. If your child is old enough to use a dry powder inhaler device, it is less likely that other children will use this inhaler because it cannot be sprayed around and has to be put in the mouth to be activated. In any case, do speak to your child's teacher about your concerns.

# *Growing out of it?*

**My 6-year-old son has asthma. Will he grow out of it?**

This must be the most asked question about asthma! Of course everyone wants the answer to be 'yes' and it is very tempting to say that all children will grow out of their asthma. Unfortunately this is not so. Without knowing more about your son's medical history we cannot say what will happen to him for sure as he grows up. However, we do know that the milder the asthma, the more likely it is that the symptoms will disappear before a child reaches puberty. Some children seem to have their asthma symptoms (cough, wheeze and breathlessness) only when they have an upper respiratory tract infection (a cold or sore throat). For them the outlook is good.

If, on the other hand, the asthma is in association with hay fever and eczema, children are more likely to continue having asthma into adulthood. Sometimes the symptoms may lessen or disappear at puberty even with these children, but they frequently come back later in adult life.

The earlier a child develops asthma and the more frequent and severe their attacks, the less chance there is of the asthma disappearing in adolescence. Reaching puberty is even more important than usual for a child with asthma. By the age of 16 only 20–25% of youngsters will have persistent symptoms.

There are undoubtedly some adults who had asthma as children and then had no symptoms for many years, only to find in later life that the asthma has returned. It is important to remember that once you have had asthma, you always have an 'asthma tendency' and the asthma can recur at any time.

**Why did my asthma return? I had it as a child but then I was free of it for many years.**

The simple answer is that we don't know. It is well recognized that asthma can return after years of not having any symptoms at all. Most often this happens to young adults who apparently 'lost' their asthma in late childhood. Most children with asthma first develop symptoms before the age of 5, but many stop having symptoms by the time they reach puberty. By their late 20s, around 25% will have frequent asthma symptoms, around 30% will have no symptoms, and the remainder will be only mildly affected by their asthma.

This is why we tend to talk about asthma going 'into remission' as young children grow, rather than being cured. We do not know exactly why this happens. The influence of body hormones at the beginning of puberty plays some part. In some cases, asthma returns in middle age or even later, as your question seems to indicate. This is even more of a mystery, though we feel sure there must be some trigger in the environment which can 'switch on' asthma that has been dormant for many years.

# *Adolescents and young adults*

**I read somewhere that children who have asthma mature
later than average. Why is this?**

Research has shown that children with asthma tend to mature
physically 1–2 years later than other children. If they have severe
or difficult asthma, this is often the case, but medicine treatment
does not seem to be the cause. X-rays of bones in children give a
good indication of maturity and, in children with asthma, *bone age*
will often be 1 or 2 years behind actual age.

The practical effect of this is most important in adolescents,
as they will have their growth spurt and their signs of puberty
later than their friends, who do not have asthma. Although we
can reassure them that they will 'catch up' later, this may be of
little comfort at a time when it is so important to them to be
the same as everybody else. Height and weight should be
measured and recorded at each asthma review. This will enable
the doctor or asthma nurse to monitor growth and reassure
both the child and their parents. The delayed growth issues
need to be handled very sensitively and concerns listened to
and acknowledged.

So, in physical terms it is true, but there is no evidence that young
people with asthma mature emotionally later than their peers.

**I'm in the middle of my GCSEs, and my asthma has got
much worse because of the pressure. I'm afraid that I
might have an attack during one of my papers. How can I
avoid this?**

All examinations cause stress and some people cope better than
others at this time. As important school exams are held in the
summer months, this brings added problems because they coincide
with the hay fever season and high pollen counts. Both of these
make asthma worse in many young people. Prevention wherever
possible is always better than cure, and there are a few things that
may help.

- April or early May is a good time to visit your doctor or asthma nurse for extra advice about your asthma control. Regular peak expiratory flow readings for a few weeks, which are recorded on a record chart, will help you find out whether your asthma is well controlled or not. If your asthma is not under good control and you are having asthma symptoms, your asthma medicines need to be reviewed by your doctor or asthma nurse. Hay fever medicines can reduce the trigger effect of pollen on the asthma, even if you do not have the obvious hay fever symptoms of sneezing, running nose and itchy eyes.

- Always make sure that you carry your reliever inhaler with you and take your preventer treatment as discussed with your doctor or asthma nurse. If you are already in the middle of your exams, and your asthma is not well controlled, you may want to ask them about a possible short course of steroid tablets to tide you over the most important exam days. If you do suffer badly from your asthma or hay fever during the exam time and you feel this has had an effect on your exam performance, a certificate or letter from your doctor or asthma nurse stating the problems you have had, may help the examiners.

- Despite your exams, make sure you have some time to enjoy a social life and activities with friends. This helps to relieve some of the tensions that you are all under and provides a good network of support. Relaxation can help to reduce the chances of having an asthma attack owing to stress.

- Ask your doctor or asthma nurse for an asthma action plan. This will help you know what to do if symptoms are troublesome. They will work out a plan with you that is right for you. This plan can be based on either asthma symptoms or peak flow reading.

**Personal action plan – things you might wish to discuss with your doctor or asthma nurse**

- How can I help keep my child's asthma under control?

- What do I do if my child's usual relief inhaler is no longer effective?

- Can you tell me what to look for so I know if my child is having an asthma attack?

- Will a peak flow meter be useful to check if my child's asthma is getting worse?

- How can I help my child if their asthma gets worse?

- After a bad asthma attack, does my child need to see the doctor or asthma nurse?

- Does my child need to see my doctor or asthma nurse for a regular check-up?

- Can I have some written instructions so I know what to do if my child has a bad asthma attack?

- How can I help my young child use a spacer and mask device with the asthma inhaler?

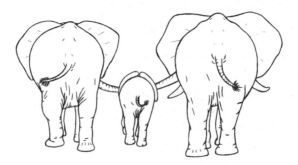

# 8
# Emergencies

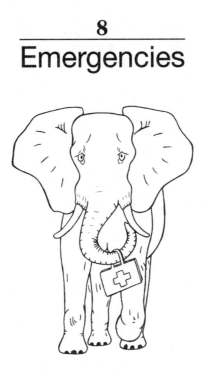

**In this chapter you will learn about:**

- how to tell when your asthma is going out of control

- the danger signs which may be present before asthma attacks

- when to worry and when to call for help

- what immediate action to take while waiting for help

- how to learn lessons from asthma attacks and to prevent them in future.

In the UK in the last 30 years, the number of hospital admissions for acute asthma has gone up dramatically, although in the last few years the rise has tailed off. This rise has been particularly noticeable in children, most of all in children under 5 years of age. Researchers have tried to understand the reasons for this. Whatever these are, there are now around 69 000 such admissions in the UK every year. We believe that nearly all of these hospital admissions represent a missed opportunity for preventive asthma treatment. If health professionals as well as people with asthma (or their carers) can improve how they recognize the early warning signs of asthma attacks, and if the right action is taken, many asthma attacks and hospital admissions can be prevented.

Throughout this book we stress the need to recognize uncontrolled asthma. Early action on your part to prevent the asthma episode from worsening is so important. The first section in this chapter deals with the early warning signs and symptoms of asthma attacks. The most important of these is the failure of symptoms to respond to your usual reliever treatment. If this is happening to you, don't accept this as just one of those things! It is a sign of potentially serious trouble and perhaps the beginning of an asthma attack.

The second section gives advice on what to do if you or someone you are with has an asthma attack. Sometimes it is important to get to hospital urgently. In this section you will learn when to call for an ambulance or make your way quickly to hospital. Although we work in the community and would like all of our patients to stay out of hospital, we believe that, for some people with uncontrolled asthma or an acute attack, it is important to get to hospital as fast as possible. Sometimes this means that you do not see your GP first. However, one of the reasons for the increase in hospital admissions for acute asthma is that perhaps too many people bypass their doctor and go straight to hospital! In this chapter, we try to help you get it right – when to worry and when to continue self-managing your asthma. The decision to 'self-refer' to hospital is one that is best part of an agreed plan between you and the hospital specialist, GP or asthma nurse (see the section on **Written action plans for asthma** in Chapter 5).

The final section deals with recovery from asthma attacks. We feel this is just as important as recognizing the early stages. Everyone with asthma is more vulnerable and may suffer a repeat episode during the weeks following an attack. It is a time when you should take a very careful note of your symptoms and peak flow readings. Do go and see your doctor or asthma nurse for an asthma check as soon as possible after an acute attack. The main reason for this is to find out if the attack could have been prevented. In particular, were you on the correct treatment and were you taking it in the right way?

If you were admitted to hospital, arrangements should have been made for you to be seen again soon after you had gone home. This might mean that you would be seen for a check-up at the hospital, or at your usual GP surgery. In either event, you should have a check-up in the 3 days after the attack.

# Symptoms and warnings

### What are the warning signs and symptoms of an asthma attack?

Most people have symptoms, like cough, wheeze or shortness of breath, for a number of days before they have an asthma attack. Sometimes these symptoms are present for a few weeks or even months without the person realizing they are due to their asthma being out of control. Many people with asthma say that they do not feel they are listened to when they consult a doctor or asthma nurse for their asthma. The reason for this may be because some health professionals are not very aware of the danger signs of asthma attacks. It may also be because the person with asthma does not explain clearly what they are worried about, or that they don't describe all their symptoms to the doctor or asthma nurse. It is therefore very important to explain that they think their symptoms may be due to uncontrolled asthma when they seek medical help. At the end of this chapter, as in all the others, we have listed some of the things you might want to discuss when you see your doctor or asthma nurse for check-ups.

Warning signs before asthma attacks vary from person to person. In one rare form of asthma, known as brittle asthma, people may go from no symptoms at all to severe acute life-threatening asthma within minutes. For most people however, there are clear warning signs. These are:

- your usual symptoms of asthma getting worse or going on for days, and not improving when you try to use your usual treatment

- changes in peak flow readings – if you monitor your own peak expiratory flow, changes in the readings are usually present before the symptoms start; these readings therefore give early warnings of an asthma attack. There are three patterns to watch out for:
  - steadily falling readings
  - morning dips
  - an increased morning to evening gap in readings. We have discussed these changes in the section on diagnosis and peak expiratory flow in Chapter 3.

- unusual symptoms which always or nearly always occur before an attack – examples of these are a tickly cough, a strange sensation in the skin (usually an itch) or in your nose, light-headedness or sickness; there are other warning symptoms and it is important for everyone to recognize their own.

Asthma attacks vary from mild to very severe. Mild attacks may only involve slight coughing, wheezing or difficulty in breathing. In a severe attack, there will be extreme difficulty in speaking and breathing. A person may become blue around the lips from shortage of oxygen (*cyanosis*). This colour can be very difficult to judge, particularly in artificial light or if you have very dark skin.

It is important to be aware that a mild attack may develop into a very severe one. This may occur suddenly or take a few days or weeks to happen. It is for this reason that all asthma attacks should be taken seriously, even if they appear to be mild. Failure of relief medication to last for 4 hours or to have its usual effect is a very important sign, both for people with asthma and for health professionals. It is very important to tell your doctor or asthma nurse if your usual medication is not helping your asthma symptoms.

**How do I tell if my asthma symptoms are serious?**

The symptoms of an attack are the same as the symptoms of asthma – these are, coughing, wheezing and difficulty in breathing. All of these symptoms may occur together, but during an acute attack, shortness of breath is usually the most noticeable. If you suddenly get worse, your asthma symptoms should improve when extra relief medication is taken. This improvement should last for at least 4 hours. Therefore, if your symptoms are getting worse and they do not improve with your usual asthma relief medication, or if they worsen again within 4 hours, then you should seek medical advice.

Someone whose asthma is well controlled should not be getting these symptoms. If you are, you probably need more or different asthma medicines. When you phone your doctor's practice, explain clearly to the receptionist what is happening. Say that your asthma is out of control and that you need to see the doctor or asthma nurse urgently. When you do go to the practice, repeat all the information to the doctor or asthma nurse, because the receptionist may not have done so.

**'Everyone' seems to know how to treat an epileptic fit or diabetic emergency, but not how to treat someone having an asthma attack. Why? Is it the fault of first aid courses which give it such a low priority? Should there be more public education?**

Asthma has had a very low profile until recent years, and very little attention has been paid to teaching people how to cope with someone having an attack. As it is one of the commonest medical conditions found in the developed world, there definitely should be more public education about it. First aid courses probably have given low priority to asthma, and we certainly hope this will change as public recognition of the importance of asthma increases.

There are excellent sources of educational material from the charity UK Asthma (formerly known as the National Asthma Campaign). In addition, Education for Health (incorporating the National Respiratory Training Centre and Heartsave), with headquarters in Warwick, provides special asthma courses for health professionals throughout the UK (addresses in *Appendix*).

### Is it right that itching is a sign of an asthma attack?

Yes. Itching often comes before an attack, more commonly in children, and mainly in the upper half of the body. If this is one of your symptoms you will find that the itching tends to occur in the same area of the body each time. It is called '*prodromal* itching' and occurs at an early stage of an asthma attack. It is usually something that children with asthma know about, although they may not complain about it. The cause is not understood, but it may be an allergic reaction. You can make use of this warning – if extra relief medication is taken when the itching first occurs, it may stop the attack.

### What is a silent chest?

When someone has an asthma attack they have increases in one or more of the common symptoms of asthma – coughing, wheezing and shortness of breath. As long as air is passing in and out of the lungs, the wheezing will stay and can be heard, and the breathing will tend to be quite noisy. However, when the air passages are so tight that very little air can get into the lungs, these symptoms are less obvious. In particular there may be no wheezing, and in this case the breathing becomes very quiet. When the doctor or asthma nurse listens with a stethoscope, no sounds of breathing are heard. This situation where someone is having difficulty getting air in and out of their lungs is described as a silent chest, and all doctors recognize it as a sign of a very severe attack. Emergency treatment is required for this condition.

# *First aid for emergencies*

If you are concerned that your asthma attack is getting very bad or if you are concerned about someone else who is having an attack, call for advice or help immediately. While waiting for help, it is important that the reliever medication is used; in high doses if necessary. This information is given in more detail in the rest of this chapter, but for people with asthma and those around them, the essential points in dealing with asthma episodes follow.

## *Action to take*

### If my chest feels very tight and my Ventolin (salbutamol) is not working, what should I do?

As we have said many times in this book, failure to obtain relief from your usual reliever, whichever one you take, is an important sign of uncontrolled asthma. An attack may be on the way, and quick action is needed. Seek medical advice urgently. In the meantime self-treatment must be continued. Even though it may not seem to be working, it is important to take your reliever in high doses until you can get other treatment. Ideally you will have discussed with your doctor or asthma nurse what to do if this situation arises, but the following will help as general guidance.

- **Emergency use of reliever inhalers**. Usually 2–6 puffs, taken one at a time and inhaled separately, every 20–30 minutes is sufficient. However if you are not getting relief, take extra puffs until the emergency services arrive. If you have a spacer device available, use this to take the medication. This way of taking your relief medicine works as well as a nebulizer and is perfectly safe when used in an emergency. Once you have taken your asthma reliever medicine, concentrate on breathing steadily, and staying relaxed. It is still important to call for help or advice, even if you do feel better.

- We would also recommend that you **start taking steroid tablets** (prednisolone) straight away if you have them available. This should be part of your action plan or self-management plan; if not, we suggest that you discuss it with your health professional. A dose of 30–60 mg (6–12 tablets) for adults and 20–30 mg (4–6 tablets) for children is usually suitable. You will need to take these tablets for several days until the attack is over.

### What is the best way for me to treat a very bad attack?

During a very bad attack it becomes difficult for you to speak, because of breathlessness. This is an emergency, which needs treatment in hospital. Take a high dose of relief medication: usually 2–6 puffs, taken one at a time, and inhaled separately, every 20–30 minutes is sufficient. Sometimes higher doses are needed and it is important to take more reliever medicine if you do not improve at all. These doses are not dangerous; in fact the equivalent of 25–50 puffs of salbutamol is the dose that is given in a nebulizer. If you have a spacer device available, use it to take your reliever through this device. The box on the next page shows Education for Health's (National Respiratory Training Centre) advice.

Otherwise, use your device as best you can, as often as you need until you feel better. Salbutamol or terbutaline should start to work within a few minutes and this is why it is always important to carry your reliever treatment with you. If it is available, take a peak expiratory flow reading before you start and make a note of the reading. Check your peak flow again after about 15 minutes to see if it has improved. This way you can see if your reliever medicine is helping.

Try to remain calm, and arrange to get to hospital. If your own doctor is with you, he or she will arrange an ambulance. If you are on your own, phone the emergency services and ask for an ambulance. Tell them your asthma is severe and that you need help urgently.

For a very bad attack a course of steroid tablets is always necessary. If you have these available, then the course should be started straight away. These tablets take approximately 6 hours to

**EMERGENCY TREATMENT**

**VIA THE SPACER DEVICE***

*The severe asthma attack: what to look for and what to do*

**Any of these signs means the attack is severe:**

1. The usual relief medication does not help.

2. The symptoms (cough, breathlessness, wheeze) get worse.

3. The patient is too breathless to speak normally.

**How to deal with the attack:**

1. Give the reliever drug.

2. Call the doctor or ambulance if the condition is not relieved in 5 minutes. If the attack is very bad, call for medical help immediately.

3. If the patient has an emergency supply of oral steroids (prednisolone; soluble prednisolone), give the stated dose as soon as possible.

*(*Taken from the National Respiratory Training Centre [now Education for Health] card)*

begin to work, and so it is important to start them promptly, particularly if you are away from home and there may be some delay in getting medical attention. Steroid tablets save lives in severe asthma attacks, and they should be used early in the attack rather than as a last resort. It is important to discuss an action plan for your asthma with your own doctor or asthma nurse when you are well, so that you are more confident about what to do if you should have such a bad attack.

**What is the best thing to do when I gasp for breath?**

It may be difficult to stay calm when you are short of breath, but this is one of the best things you can do. Overbreathing (or hyperventilation) as a result of panic will make an asthma attack worse. Try to slow down your breathing by taking 5–10 seconds to breathe in and 5–10 seconds to breathe out. Relaxation exercises include practice at breathing slowly and regularly, and are good preparation for dealing with asthma attacks. Ask the doctor or asthma nurse at your clinic for more information about these.

As well as trying to relax as best you can, take frequent doses of your reliever treatment until you start to feel relief, as described in the previous question. If this doesn't work, then you must seek urgent medical assistance.

**Can I go straight to hospital if I have an attack?**

Yes you can, and it may be the best step for you to take if you suffer from sudden severe asthma attacks. If you are one of those few people whose asthma is bad enough to require several hospital admissions each year, then you will be under specialist care – or should be. Usually you will have instructions as to when it is best to go direct to hospital. For most people with asthma this is not the case, and the majority of asthma attacks can be managed without the need for hospital admission. Your GP and asthma nurse are likely to be familiar with your asthma, and in a good position to help deal with acute attacks. There has not been much research on how asthma attacks are treated in the community. One national study during the early 1990s showed that only one out of every seven people with acute attacks of asthma in the community was admitted to hospital.

**How do we know when to take our child to hospital?**

In emergencies there are two options open to you for medical help. The first is to contact your general practice, and this is what we would suggest in most situations. In certain circumstances it may be better to go straight to hospital. If your child has had a number

of admissions to hospital for acute asthma, then it is best to agree
with the specialist at the hospital what to do. This is called an 'open
door policy', and it means that, if your child has a bad attack which
is not responding to an agreed treatment plan, you can take him
or her direct to the hospital ward, without contacting your GP first.
This is best for children who have repeated admissions for asthma,
and for adults with 'brittle asthma' whose attacks come on rapidly
and can be very severe. For most other people with asthma, it is
usually best to see a doctor or asthma nurse who knows you and
your child's history.

GPs in the National Health Service provide emergency cover
during the working day; however, under new arrangements, many
do not do so after normal working hours. In most parts of the UK,
emergency care is provided either by cooperatives run by local
GPs or by the Primary Care Organizations. During normal hours,
your practice will be able to manage most asthma attacks without
the need for hospital admission, but if admission is needed, it is
generally better for your doctor or asthma nurse to arrange this
and for you to go to hospital with a referral letter from the practice,
unless of course you are extremely unwell, when an ambulance is
best. If your GP cannot be contacted, it is safer to go straight to
hospital.

**Most asthma attacks may be prevented by taking regular
asthma medicines as advised, by having regular check-ups
with a health professional and by following an agreed asthma
action plan.**

For uncontrolled asthma outside normal working hours, the
services provided by GPs and the Primary Care Organizations are
more appropriate for most people than are Accident and Emergency
departments.

When asthma is diagnosed there are three questions which
should be answered to your satisfaction by your doctor or asthma
nurse:

- What should I do in an attack?

- How do I contact a doctor in an emergency?

- When should I go straight to the hospital?

If you haven't covered these questions with your doctor or asthma nurse (or have forgotten the answers!) then go over them when you next have the opportunity.

Most people's asthma is not so severe that immediate treatment at the hospital is required. It is much better for you to have guidance from your GP in advance of any problem, rather than afterwards. **Many people with uncontrolled asthma symptoms wait far too long before contacting their practice. If your usual asthma medicine is not helping, or if you are getting increasing symptoms of cough, wheeze or shortness of breath, see or speak to your usual GP or asthma nurse as soon as you can. However, in a severe attack, go to the hospital first.**

### Sometimes repeat doses of my reliever inhaler do not have any effect. What shall I do?

This is potentially serious! Failure to get a useful benefit from repeat doses of a reliever is the most important sign of uncontrolled asthma. You should get help urgently and, if you have a short course of steroid tablets prescribed for this purpose, you should start these immediately, as well as taking extra reliever medication. If you have an asthma action plan (self-management plan; see Chapter 5) that has been previously agreed with your doctor or asthma nurse, then this should contain guidance on what to do. Otherwise you should get medical advice as soon as possible.

### Can a child die of asthma?

Yes. Such tragedies are very rare but do occur. Of the approximately 1500 deaths from asthma which occur each year in the UK, only 1–2% are in the under-14 age group (around 15–30 deaths per year). To put this into perspective, remember that 10–15% of children suffer from asthma; so out of the million or so children with asthma there are very few fatal attacks.

Unfortunately some asthma deaths cannot be prevented. They result from sudden unexpected fatal attacks, nearly always against a background of very severe asthma or allergy (e.g. peanut allergy). Anyone with a previously diagnosed severe food allergy **and** asthma should have an emergency kit available. This kit should be in addition to the usual asthma medication. This kit includes a special adrenaline injection (Epipen or Anapen), a course of steroid tablets and a course of antihistamine tablets.

A fatal asthma attack is exceptionally rare in a previously healthy child. We would like to be completely reassuring on this point, but tragedies do happen. People with asthma must always be cautious if an attack of asthma seems different in some way from previous episodes, or is unresponsive to reliever treatment.

**What if I have an attack and I have no medication?**

Ideally, this should not happen. Asthma attacks can occur without warning, and so you should always try to ensure that you have some relief medication available, wherever you are. If, however, you have an attack and no medication is available, take steps to obtain treatment straight away, either from your GP, or from the nearest hospital if your symptoms are severe.

In the UK you are able to obtain an emergency supply of your asthma treatment from a local pharmacist. You will need to give some details about your asthma as well as pay for the medicines. You will pay the actual cost of the medicines as well as a dispensing fee, as the medicines are not being obtained on a prescription. Obtaining your asthma medicines in this way is only for exceptional situations. You should take care not to run out of any regular medicines and should obtain a prescription before this happens.

If the attack occurs when you are **away from home** and in the UK, emergency treatment is available from any GP working in the National Health Service. However, if you have a **severe attack**, we would always recommend hospital as the first choice. If you are in doubt about how severe your attack is (and it can be difficult), always be on the safe side and seek advice about your asthma at the hospital.

If you are abroad and do not have your asthma medication with you, we would advise you to go directly to hospital if at all possible. In an untreated attack, delay can be serious and on some occasions has been fatal. In some countries, it is possible to get a reliever inhaler (Ventolin is well known) from a pharmacy without a prescription. This will be helpful while trying to find local medical help.

**My friend has asthma. What do I do if I am with her and she has an asthma attack?**

If your friend is distressed and having difficulty breathing, this is a potentially severe attack.

- Stay calm.

- First, as in the case of any medical emergency, call for an ambulance immediately – or ask someone else to do so, if possible. Then you can start helping.

- Ask her if she has her reliever inhaler (Ventolin or terbutaline) with her. If she has, help her to take large doses of the reliever inhaler as best as she can – usually 2–6 puffs, taken one after the other. This can be repeated every 20–30 minutes (or more frequently if there is no effect). Tell her to take more if necessary while waiting for help.

- If she is struggling to use her inhaler, you can help her by making an emergency spacer device using a piece of paper rolled into a cone, or by making a hole in the bottom of a paper or polystyrene coffee cup (see Figure 8.1). Hold the cone in front of her face, and fire the inhaler 2–6 times, with about 10–15 seconds between each puff, so that she can breathe the spray via the cone or cup. Use more if she is not improving, and repeat this every few minutes while waiting for help. It is safe to do this, and it will nearly always bring some temporary relief. You won't be able to do this for the dry powder devices, but you can give repeated doses without any risk of overdose.

**Should I consult a doctor before administering Ventolin nebulizer to my son with asthma?**

Since there are no dangers from using a single dose in this way, it is probably better that you start treatment immediately and then

**Figure 8.1** In an emergency, high doses of reliever bronchodilator medication should be used while waiting for help. Ideally, the metered dose inhaler should be used with a spacer device (*right*). If no spacer is available, a paper coffee cup (*below*) with a hole cut in the base or a piece of paper rolled up into a funnel will do.

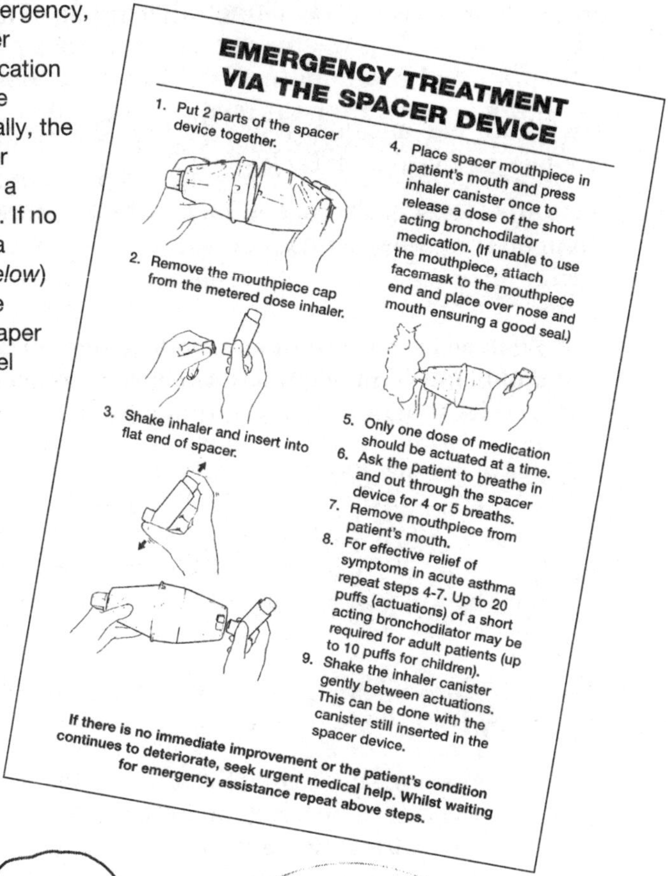

EMERGENCY TREATMENT VIA THE SPACER DEVICE

1. Put 2 parts of the spacer device together.

2. Remove the mouthpiece cap from the metered dose inhaler.

3. Shake inhaler and insert into flat end of spacer.

4. Place spacer mouthpiece in patient's mouth and press inhaler canister once to release a dose of the short acting bronchodilator medication. (If unable to use the mouthpiece, attach facemask to the mouthpiece end and place over nose and mouth ensuring a good seal.)

5. Only one dose of medication should be actuated at a time.

6. Ask the patient to breathe in and out through the spacer device for 4 or 5 breaths.

7. Remove mouthpiece from patient's mouth.

8. For effective relief of symptoms in acute asthma repeat steps 4-7. Up to 20 puffs (actuations) of a short acting bronchodilator may be required for adult patients (up to 10 puffs for children).

9. Shake the inhaler canister gently between actuations. This can be done with the canister still inserted in the spacer device.

If there is no immediate improvement or the patient's condition continues to deteriorate, seek urgent medical help. Whilst waiting for emergency assistance repeat above steps.

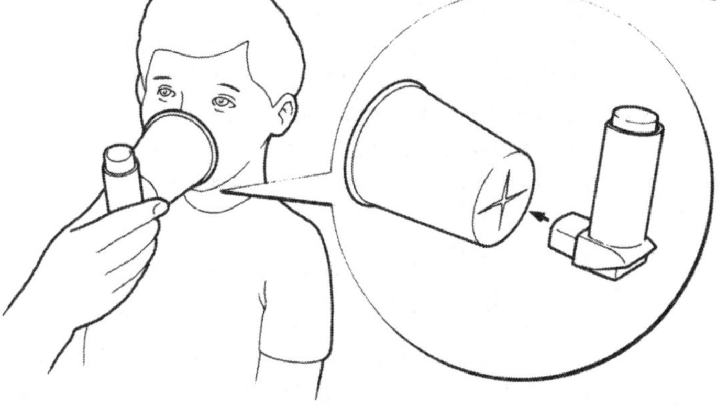

call the doctor or ambulance service, depending on the circumstances. This treatment may be life saving in a severe attack. The potential problem in doing this does not come from the nebulizer, or even from the medicine in the nebulizer. The danger comes from **not recognizing** when asthma is getting worse, and from **not** doing enough. We would advise that a short course of steroid tablets is also needed whenever an attack is bad enough to need treatment with a nebulizer. So, even if your son is a lot better after the treatment, he should still see a doctor or asthma nurse urgently – within a few hours if possible.

If he needs a nebulizer for an attack, this is because his asthma is out of control. If the nebulizer relieves the symptoms for at least 4 hours, then his attack has responded to the treatment, and he should continue with his self-management (or action) plan. However, if this does not happen, it is important that other treatment should be obtained. We now know that a spacer device works as well as a nebulizer in most cases of acute asthma so long as high doses of reliever medicine are used, i.e. equivalent to the dose that is given by nebulizer.

**My sister has asthma. How can I help her if she starts to hyperventilate?**

Hyperventilation (or overbreathing) means breathing more rapidly than is necessary or than is good for someone. It occurs commonly in people who are anxious or frightened (whatever the reason), and causes symptoms of light-headedness, feeling sick, and tingling in the hands and feet and around the lips. For someone with an asthma attack, who is trying desperately to breathe, it is an understandable reaction. Anything that helps to slow down her breathing will help your sister, including a gentle and calm approach by those around her. Extra use of her reliever medication will help to improve the asthma attack and this, hopefully, should reduce her hyperventilation.

The well-known trick of breathing in and out of a paper bag is less helpful in asthma than in other circumstances. There is already a shortage of oxygen, and this may be made worse by breathing in used air from a bag. It will be more useful to talk slowly and reassuringly to your sister in order to slow down her rate of breathing.

### How bad does an attack have to be before seeking medical advice?

Everyone's asthma is different, and so the detailed answer to this question depends a lot on the features of your own asthma. Past experience is often helpful in deciding whether you need help. Ideally you and everyone else should have a personal action or self-management plan for treating asthma episodes (see the section on *Written action plans for asthma* in Chapter 5). When your asthma goes out of control, you follow the plan. If your symptoms fail to improve, it is a sign that you need medical advice. Severe symptoms mean that you must call for medical help straight away. Here are some examples of symptoms that are severe:

- difficulty in speaking, or not being able to complete sentences in one breath

- severe difficulty in breathing

- blue discoloration of the lips or tongue

- a very fast pulse (more than 120 per minute in an adult or more than 140 per minute in a child)

- a very fast breathing rate (more than 25 per minute in an adult, more than 40 in children aged 5–15 years and more than 50 per minute in preschool children)

- becoming exhausted by the attack

- a peak flow reading less than half the usual level.

If you are unsure, it is always better and safer to seek advice early in an asthma attack, rather than later. The worse your asthma attack is when you ask for help, the more difficult it is to treat.

**How soon should I have a check-up after an asthma attack?**

After you have had an asthma attack or episode of uncontrolled asthma you should see your doctor or asthma nurse within 2 or 3 days. We use the terms 'asthma attack' or 'uncontrolled asthma' to mean that your asthma was out of control and that:

- you needed to use extra reliever medication (either by an inhaler or through a nebulizer), or

- you needed a short course of steroid tablets, or

- you needed to be seen as an emergency for asthma either by the GP out of hours service or the Accident and Emergency department, or

- you were admitted to hospital for asthma.

A check-up is very important for a number of reasons. This will give you an opportunity to discuss why you had the attack and what could have been done to prevent the attack. You can also find out how you can prevent any future attacks. Your doctor or asthma nurse will probably do this in two ways. They will:

- make sure that you understand how and when to take your medication, and

- agree a personal action or self-management plan with you or change your plan if you already have one (see the section on *Written action plans for asthma* in Chapter 5).

Asthma UK has produced two useful booklets called *After your asthma attack* and *After your child's asthma attack*, which contain useful information. They are both available from Asthma UK (see *Appendix*).

**Why am I always sick after an asthma attack?**

The sickness may be part of the attack, as vomiting is a symptom of asthma in some people. Nausea or 'sickness' may be one of your early symptoms of attacks. The vomit often contains a lot of mucus or slimy liquid. The attack may be mild to severe and sometimes causes a severe loss of fluid (*dehydration*) with the need for hospital admission. Because this symptom is uncommon, the diagnosis of asthma may be delayed. The clues to diagnosing asthma are usually present at the end of the attack, when the vomiting lessens. The more common symptoms of shortness of breath and wheezing tend to be present at this stage.

Oxygen shortage during attacks is another possible explanation for vomiting. Asthma attacks cause narrowing of the airways, which means air cannot get through to the lungs very easily. This can cause a shortage of oxygen in the blood, which may result in a feeling of sickness. A similar thing happens when people (with or without asthma) go up to high altitudes and develop 'altitude' or 'mountain' sickness.

**For how long do I need to continue a higher dose of my inhalers after I have had a cold?**

This is another of those situations which is different for each person; there is no rule that would work for everyone. You are doing the right thing by increasing your medication when an important trigger factor, such as a cold, comes along. The trigger makes the airways hyperreactive or twitchy, and this may lead to a bad attack of asthma. It is wise to try to prevent this by increasing the use of relief medication as well as the preventer (if you usually take both of these).

If you are taking one of the combination asthma inhalers, Symbicort in particular, some recent research suggests that this may be used four to five times a day when your symptoms flare up. Symbicort contains a long-acting reliever (formoterol) and a preventer (budesonide).

Standard advice for increasing the dose of preventer with colds etc. has changed recently. Rather than doubling the dose, which may be effective for some people, successful control is more likely to be re-established if you increase your dosage by four to five times the usual dose. This should be continued until you are feeling better and your peak flow readings have come back to their normal levels. Once the symptoms have cleared up, the

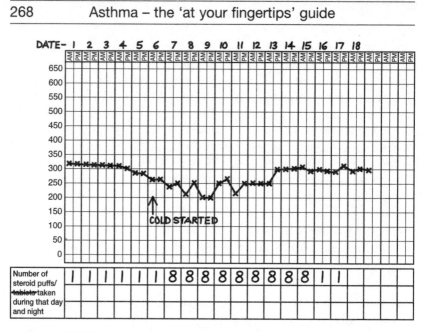

**Figure 8.2** This is the chart of a boy whose asthma went out of control following a cold. He increased his inhaled steroid preventer according to his asthma action plan.

twitchiness of the air passages has probably settled. A rule of thumb is to continue on the higher dose for 2 weeks after the start of the episode; then the dose of preventer can be reduced to your previous level. This method often works well but it is not always suitable for everyone.

The best way to tell if your asthma has improved after an attack is to keep a peak flow diary chart, which gives a more accurate picture of when the asthma episode is over. Figure 8.2 shows the chart of a boy whose asthma went out of control following a cold. It is clear from looking at the chart when his asthma returned to normal. This method is best because it helps in two ways:

- It ensures that you take enough extra medicine, because the dose can be increased until the readings improve to your normal level and settle.

- Once your readings have settled at your normal level, and are not changing much from day to day, you can then reduce the dose. If you continue to keep your diary, you will be able to increase your asthma medicines again if your asthma deteriorates.

This approach ensures you take sufficient medication when you need it and also that you do not take more asthma medicines than necessary (see Figure 8.3).

Normally your readings should be about the same whenever they are taken, but if your airways are twitchy, they will vary by more than 20% from morning to evening (see Figure 8.3).

We give more detail about using your chart to decide when it is safe to reduce your dose to its normal level, in the section on **Written action plans for Asthma** in Chapter 5.

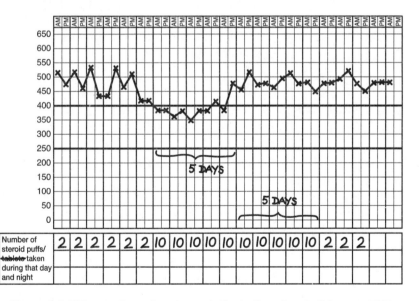

**Figure 8.3** If the readings drop towards the bottom line, in this case 50% of best, then decisive action is needed. This person has followed his action plan which advised him to increase his preventer inhaler to five times the usual dose, 10 puffs a day, until he was better.

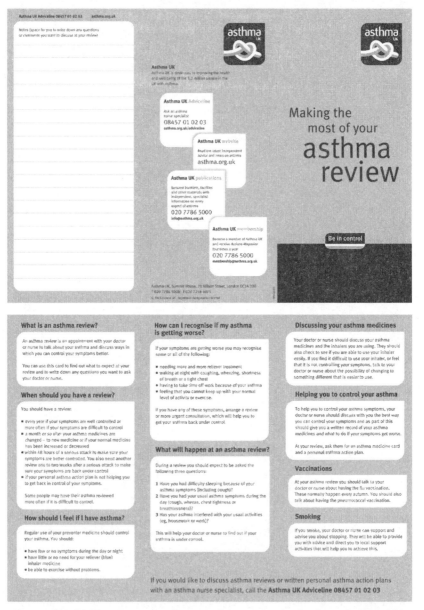

**Figure 8.4** *Making the most of your asthma review* leaflet from Asthma UK.

(Courtesy of Asthma UK.)

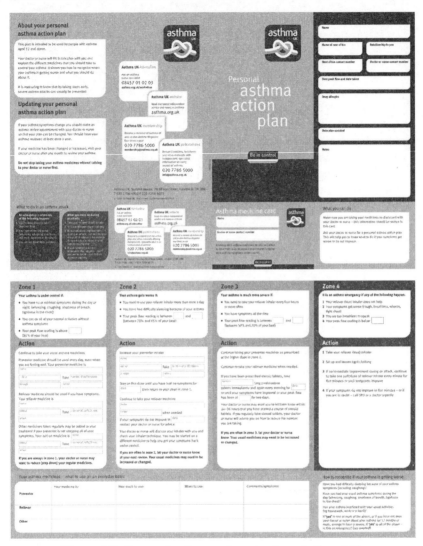

**Figure 8.5** *Personal asthma action plan* from Asthma UK.

(Courtesy of Asthma UK.)

**Personal action plan – things you might wish to discuss
with your doctor or asthma nurse**

In this chapter you learnt how to tell if you are going to have an asthma attack, what to do if your symptoms get worse or if you do have an attack, what to do after an asthma attack or after an episode of uncontrolled asthma. The most important thing is that you should see your doctor or asthma nurse for a check-up within 3 days of having an asthma attack.

When you go for this check-up, it will be helpful if you take your medicines with you. These can be checked to see that you have the right medicines and that your inhaler technique is satisfactory. Poor inhaler technique is a common reason for asthma medicines not working properly. If you are recording your peak flow readings, take them with you so they can be discussed with your asthma doctor or nurse.

During your check-up you might want to ask the following questions:

- Why did my asthma go out of control?
- Am I on the right asthma medicine?
- Do I use my inhaler correctly?
- What are the danger signs of uncontrolled asthma?
- Should I have an emergency supply of steroid tablets in case my asthma goes out of control? How do I know when to take these?
- How can I make sure that I get emergency help next time this happens?
- Do I need to change my personal action (self-management) plan?

Asthma UK has developed an asthma review card (see Figures 8.4–8.5). This sets out what you should expect from an asthma review with your doctor or asthma nurse and will help you to ask the right questions. It is available free of charge from Asthma UK or from their website (see *Appendix* for this).

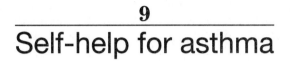

# 9
# Self-help for asthma

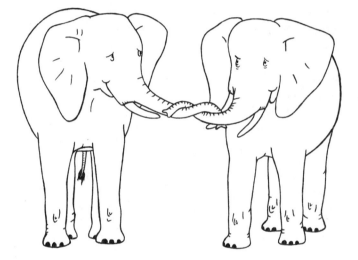

We hope that we have written enough in this book to convince you that your role in managing your asthma is extremely important. Treatment is a partnership between you, your doctor and asthma nurse and you have every right to be involved with your treatment, and to question and disagree with management decisions. However, we want you to have the right information because this will help you decide what is best for you and your asthma.

Information is much more readily available now in comparison with a few years ago. Computers are everywhere, and access to the internet has become quicker and less expensive. As a result access to information is instantaneous from almost anywhere in the world. However, it is important to be aware that much of this information may be inaccurate and unreliable. It is best to visit recommended websites. When you discuss something you are concerned about with the doctor or asthma nurse, you may have already searched and obtained information yourself.

## *Asthma charities*

The patient charity the National Asthma Campaign changed its name in 2004 to Asthma UK and is the largest charity working solely for people with asthma (see the question below). Each year it gives around £3 million to a variety of research projects. Another patient charity, the British Lung Foundation, is also involved in raising awareness of not only asthma, but other respiratory conditions as well. It also funds research projects.

Only a small proportion of people with asthma are involved with self-help groups. Some people feel that they focus too much attention on asthma, rather than encouraging a positive attitude to ignore it, and carry on regardless. We have some sympathy, but disagree. The aim of the asthma charities is to help people live their lives to the full, preferably with minimal interference from their asthma.

Try to support the work of the asthma charities as much as possible, by joining in on activities and events, and by helping to raise money for them. The research they fund may find a cure and be the breakthrough we are all wanting. Your contribution is vital and you can play an important part.

Addresses of the charities are given in the *Appendix*.

### Is there an asthma charity and if so, how can we help?

The main asthma charity in the UK is Asthma UK (formerly called the National Asthma Campaign). It was formed in 1990 by the merger of two smaller charities – the Asthma Research Council, and the Asthma Society and Friends of the Asthma Research Council. You can help by joining as a member (an application form is provided in the back of this book). You pay a small subscription fee and you will receive a quarterly magazine, which will keep you informed about important issues related to asthma.

There are two other charities that raise large sums of money for research into asthma: the British Lung Foundation was formed in 1985, and supports adults and children with all kinds of lung disorders and conditions; and the Chest, Heart and Stroke Associations in Scotland and Northern Ireland have a long tradition of supporting patients with chest illness.

Allergy UK is a charity dedicated to improving the lives of people with allergy, and of course asthma also falls into that category; we have provided details of this charity as well as the Anaphylaxis Campaign in the *Appendix*.

Many people support Asthma UK and the British Lung Foundation by taking part in sponsored events such as the London Marathon. Not only does exercise keep you fit, but these events are also fun, with an enormous amount of public support, even if they are hard work and require a committed training programme! This valuable support raises the awareness of the charities, and in addition large amounts of money are pledged and given to support the charities in their work. If you are interested in running to support these charities please contact them directly.

### Are there any groups where I can get sympathy and understanding?

Asthma UK at present has only a few local branches, but there are still ways of getting understanding, advice and support. Asthma UK's Adviceline is run by specially trained asthma nurses. This telephone line is open Monday to Friday from 9.00 am to 5.00 pm (telephone number 08457 01 02 03; calls are charged at local rates). There is also an email adviceline accessed via the main website (see *Appendix*). Asthma UK has offices in London, Edinburgh, Cardiff and Belfast.

Asthma UK has excellent booklets and information sheets, obtainable direct from the charity or via its website. In addition, frequently asked questions are posted on the website in a number of different languages.

The British Lung Foundation has a network of support groups throughout the UK called Breathe Easy and has recently established Baby Breathe Easy groups. Their website has all the contact details for these groups and there is an email enquiry service. The British Lung Foundation also has excellent booklets and information sheets. The Chest, Heart and Stroke Associations have an advice line in Northern Ireland and an email service in Scotland (see *Appendix* for all this information).

Some general practices have special times set aside for people with asthma to meet together, and to be able to ask advice from a GP or asthma nurse. In addition some practices have Expert Patient Groups. Ask your local practice what services are available locally.

# Information about asthma

### Is there a video about asthma I can understand?

Videos on asthma are less available nowadays because internet websites have taken over as a way of providing information. Some people like to watch video clips about asthma as well as read books and leaflets. Asthma UK's website shows video clips on inhaler devices as well as a fun section especially for children (see *Appendix*).

### Is there any literature available that is easy to understand?

Yes, this book for example! Asthma UK also has some of the best asthma information around, which is easy to read and understandable. Their excellent series of leaflets are constantly being reviewed and updated. Many pharmaceutical companies also produce excellent booklets for adults and children. Nearly all GPs' surgeries, pharmacists and hospital outpatient departments hold stocks of a wide range of these leaflets.

Asthma UK leaflets can be downloaded from their website as well (see *Appendix* for address).

**Is there anywhere I can call about asthma where they might speak other languages?**

Asthma UK has a new multilingual advice service. This service is available through the Asthma UK Adviceline to help people whose first language is not English discuss their concerns about asthma. Callers can speak to an asthma nurse specialist via an interpreter. This service is available at the same local rates as a standard call to the Adviceline and is confidential; 150 languages are available (see *Appendix* for further information).

**Are there any information leaflets that are in languages other than English?**

Information sheets on asthma are available at Asthma UK in the following 18 languages: Arabic, Bengali, Cantonese, French, Gujurati, Hindi, Italian, Korean, Kurdish, Polish, Portuguese, Punjabi, Somali, Spanish, Tamil, Turkish, Urdu and Welsh. Other languages may be added at a later date.

**How can I find out about occupational asthma?**

The Health and Safety Executive (HSE) has a website with advice on how to identify and reduce occupational asthma. It is aimed at employers, safety representatives and health professionals and is part of a government campaign to reduce occupational asthma by 30% by 2010. The website sets out the main causes and symptoms of occupational asthma, what employers are required to do to protect their employees and how the problems are being tackled (see *Appendix*).

**My eyesight is poor and I am registered as partially sighted. I've heard that I can get Braille labels for my peak flow meter. Is that true?**

Clement Clarke International, makers of Mini-Wright peak flow meters, used to produce self-adhesive labels for their own brand of meters suitable for use by visually impaired people like you.

These labels were not available for other makes of peak flow meters. The labels used high-visibility colours of black on yellow and the raised markings created tactile graduations. The labels were carefully stuck on top of the peak flow meter scale and enabled the readings to be interpreted. Clement Clarke no longer produces these labels routinely, but current information from the company indicates they could be produced again if there was a demand. It may be worth contacting Clement Clarke directly if you need more information.

**I am registered blind and find it difficult to identify my different inhalers. Do any have Braille markings on them?**

You don't say what devices you are using, but it certainly can be a problem for you. Only a few pharmaceutical companies have markings on their inhaler devices that make them easily recognized. All Turbohaler inhaler devices (made by AstraZeneca) have Braille markings on their inhaler base, but of course not everyone can read Braille. GlaxoSmithKline produce pressurized metered dose inhalers that have raised markings on their plastic canister holders, although they are not Braille markings.

The Royal National Institute for the Blind sell different coloured raised labels called Bumpons, which you could attach to inhalers to help identify them more easily (see *Appendix*).

Another way of identifying your inhaler medicines more easily is to have different types of inhalers for each medicine, but you need to be able to tell when the device is empty. Speak with your doctor or asthma nurse for their suggestions and help.

Some inhaler devices use the colours red and green as identification markers, such as the base of the Oxis or Symbicort Turbohaler and the indicator on the Novolizer, which tells you if you breathe in correctly. If you are red/green colour blind you need to be aware of this. Again, talk to your asthma nurse or doctor to see if they can offer some practical suggestions for you.

**My asthma nurse talks about asthma guidelines. What are they and can I get information on them?**

Yes you can access them. Have a look at the British Thoracic Society (BTS) or the Scottish Intercollegiate Guideline Network (SIGN) websites (see *Appendix*). These guidelines were developed by the BTS and SIGN with input from a number of other organizations; they are updated fairly frequently and based on the best research evidence about how to diagnose, investigate and manage asthma – an essential guide for any health professional.

There are also guidelines on inhaler devices used for children. There are two guidelines – one for under-5s, the other for children aged 5–15. These can be obtained via the web from the National Institute of Health and Clinical Excellence (NICE).

**What sort of thing should happen when I go for an asthma review at the surgery?**

An asthma review is an opportunity to check how well controlled your asthma is. The Asthma UK leaflet called *How To Make the Most of your Asthma Review* is helpful. It is available via the Asthma UK website.

The questions in the box below will help you to find out how

---

**According to the UK asthma guidelines (BTS/SIGN), key questions you should expect to be asked at your asthma review are:**

1. Have you had difficulty sleeping because of your asthma symptoms (including cough)?

2. Have you had your usual asthma symptoms during the day – cough, wheeze, chest tightness or breathlessness?

3. Has your asthma interfered with your usual activities (e.g. housework, work or school)?

*(Courtesy of Royal College of Physicians)*

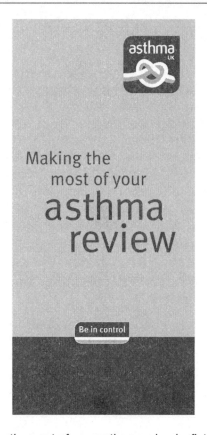

**Figure 9.1** *Making the most of your asthma review* leaflet from Asthma UK.
(Courtesy of Asthma UK.)

well controlled your asthma is. Your inhaler technique will be checked to see if you are able to use your inhaler correctly, because some devices are less easy to use than others. Ask for an asthma action plan (see Chapter 5) because it is helpful to have a reminder of what asthma medicines to take and when. Blank asthma action plans are available from Asthma UK's website (see *Appendix*) or from your doctor or asthma nurse.

Write down the things that you want to ask your doctor or asthma nurse about and take the list with you. It's very easy to forget things once you are at the practice.

**I am a teacher. How can I find information on asthma at school?**

Asthma UK has produced a school pack, which provides information on asthma for schools. They have developed a school asthma policy document to adapt for your school. It is available via the website or by post (see *Appendix*). Information on asthma at school is also available from: *www.teachernet.gov.uk/wholeschool/ healthandsafety/medical/*

General information on asthma is available from Asthma UK (see *Appendix*).

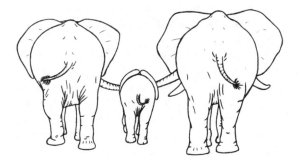

# Glossary

**acute** Short lasting. In medical terms this usually means lasting for hours or days, rather than for weeks or months.

**adrenal glands** Important glands in the body, which produce a number of hormones to control the body systems. Cortisol and cortisone are two very important examples, and adrenalin is another.

**airways** When we breathe in and out, air has to travel through hundreds of branching tubes, or airways, to and from the lung tissue (see Figure 1.1). In asthma the problem lies with these airways, which become narrow, preventing air from moving freely in and out of the lungs.

**allergens** If you are 'allergic' to something, allergens are the tiny particles or substances to which you react when you come into contact with them.

**allergic reaction** This is what happens when you come into contact with something to which you are allergic. The allergic reaction varies from person to person and according to which part of your body reacts. For example, with grass pollen, an allergic reaction may take place in the lining of your nose (in which case you get hay fever), in the airways (causing asthma symptoms) or in the skin (causing urticaria, which is similar to nettle rash).

**allergy** To have an allergy means to overreact to something in a harmful way when you come into contact with it. If you have an allergy to grass pollen you will have streaming eyes and nose, and sneezing if you come into contact with it (hay fever). Someone who is not allergic to grass pollen will not even notice grass pollen when they are in contact with it.

**alternative therapies** See **complementary therapies**.

**alveoli** These are the microscopic air spaces in the lungs which we refer to as the lung tissue. The airways get smaller and smaller as they divide into thousands of very tiny branches, and at the end of each of the smallest airways is an alveolus. Air mixes with the blood in the alveoli, and oxygen is taken in and carbon dioxide is passed out.

**aminophylline** Generic name for one of the reliever type of drugs. Aminophylline can be taken by mouth, or given by injection. There is no inhaled form. They are used less often nowadays.

**anabolic steroids** Anabolic steroids are **not** used in the treatment of asthma. They cause the body to build up muscle, and because of this have been taken by some athletes to improve performance and strength. They should not be confused with corticosteroids, which are used to treat asthma and a number of other medical conditions.

**anaphylaxis (anaphylactic attack)** A sudden, severe, potentially life-threatening allergic reaction caused, for example, by exposure to certain foods, insect stings or medicines. Symptoms include an itchy rash (hives), swelling (especially of the lips and face), difficulty breathing, either because of swelling of the throat or a severe asthma attack, vomiting, diarrhoea, cramps and low blood pressure. An anaphylactic reaction should never be ignored and the emergency services should always be called.

**anti-inflammatory drugs** These are drugs having an action against inflammation. Many diseases or conditions of the body – from asthma to arthritis to bowel disease – result in inflammation. Anti-inflammatory drugs reduce this inflammation and help the body to keep functioning as normal.

**asthma register** This is a list kept of people with asthma, usually by a general practice. All practices have a list of patients registered with them. A proportion of those will have asthma, and they are listed in a separate register. This has advantages, the most important of which is that the practice can organize its care for those with asthma, keeping a check on treatments, and how often to review people.

**atopic or atopy** To be 'atopic' is to have an allergic constitution. This means that in your make-up is the tendency to develop allergic, or atopic, conditions. The most important atopic conditions are hay fever and eczema. Asthma is strongly associated with atopy.

**beta-agonists** (also called beta-2-agonists, beta-stimulants or beta-2 stimulants). There are several names for this group of drugs, and this can be very confusing! Beta-agonists are the most important group of reliever drugs, and they include Ventolin (salbutamol) and Bricanyl (terbutaline). Most often they are taken by the inhaled route, but they can also be given in tablet, medicine or injection form. Another group of beta-agonists – the long-acting beta-agonists – include the longer-acting reliever salmeterol (Serevent) and formoterol (Oxis and Foradil).

**beta-blockers** These are very important drugs that may be used to treat high blood pressure, angina, anxiety, glaucoma and a number of other conditions. They have directly the opposite action to the beta-agonists, so they are of no help to people with asthma, and can be dangerous. Nobody with asthma should take beta-blockers, even in the form of eye drops, e.g. timolol (also known as Timoptol).

**bone age** As children grow, their bones grow with them (of course). As they grow, distinct changes can be traced in the bones by X-ray. If, for example, a child aged 7 years has an X-ray of the wrist, certain changes can be seen, which correspond to that age. In some children the bone age, as judged by X-rays, is ahead of or behind their actual age. This may be important in deciding whether a child's growth is being affected by a disease, or by certain medical treatments.

**brand names** All drugs in medicine have two names: their generic name, which is their true drug name; and a brand name under which they are sold by their manufacturer. For example, Aspro, Anadin and Disprin are all brand names of the drug aspirin.

**breath-activated inhaler** This is a type of inhaler device in which the drug is released only when a person breathes in. If no breath is taken, no drug is released from the device.

**brittle asthma** This is a severe variety of asthma and is not very common. Anyone with asthma might suffer an attack that comes on very quickly. However, people with brittle asthma can change, within minutes, from having no symptoms at all to having a very severe attack, despite taking regular treatment. Their attacks can prove very resistant to treatment. People with brittle asthma often need repeated hospital admissions, and very intensive treatment.

**bronchi and bronchioles** Bronchi are the main branches of the breathing tube (respiratory) system, taking air in and out of the lungs (see **airways**). Each time they branch, the diameter of the airway becomes smaller. The very smallest branches of the system are called bronchioles, and they end in air spaces called alveoli.

**bronchial hyperreactivity** (also called bronchial hyperresponsiveness or BHR) This means an oversensitivity in the airways, so that when the airways come into contact with irritants (e.g. allergens, smoke, viruses) they overreact in a way that causes them to produce symptoms such as coughing and wheezing.

**bronchiolitis** An important chest infection occurring in babies, usually in the winter months. It is caused by a virus, usually the respiratory syncitial virus (RSV), and often leaves the baby with coughing and wheezing for months or years afterwards.

**bronchitis** This is a very common chest infection. The main symptom is cough, with the production of phlegm (sputum), usually yellow or green in colour. It may also cause wheezing and shortness of breath, and so can be confused with asthma. Acute bronchitis can occur in any age group at any time. Chronic bronchitis is a more serious condition of older people, usually smokers or those who have lived for years in polluted atmospheres.

**bronchodilators** A medical term for relievers. They are called bronchodilators because they open up (dilate) the airways (bronchi). There are three main groups of bronchodilators, of which the beta-agonists (which include Ventolin [salbutamol] and Bricanyl [terbutaline]) are the most important.

**candida infection** Another name for **thrush** ( a fungal infection).

**cardiac asthma** This book is about bronchial asthma. Cardiac asthma is a different condition resulting from heart failure. In heart failure, fluid becomes trapped in the lungs because the heart cannot pump strongly enough to clear it. The symptoms include shortness of breath and wheezing, as with bronchial asthma, but their cause (and treatment) is completely different. Cardiac asthma is not a term used very often these days, which is just as well, since it can be confusing.

**chronic** In strictly medical terms, chronic means 'long lasting' or 'persistent'. In everyday use, many people using the word chronic mean severe or extreme. Both may apply. For example, chronic bronchitis by definition is persistent, but it often is severe.

**chronic obstructive pulmonary disease (COPD)** This is a disease of the lungs that affects people over the age of 35 and is almost always due to smoking. Sometimes it is difficult to tell if someone has COPD or asthma. Spirometry is a test that may be helpful in diagnosis of these people.

**complementary therapies** Non-medical treatments that may be taken alongside conventional drug treatments. In the past they were often referred to as 'alternative therapies', but this term suggests that the therapy is taken instead of, rather than alongside conventional medicines. Popular complementary therapies include homoeopathy, acupuncture, osteopathy and chiropractic.

**corticosteroids** This is a group of chemicals produced naturally by the body (mainly in the adrenal glands) and also synthetically as drugs. They are vital for the body's own action against infection and stress; and in disease, when given as drugs, they are among the most effective agents available to doctors to treat inflammation. So, in asthma, which is a result of inflammation in the lining of the airways, they are the most effective treatment available.

**cortisol or cortisone** A corticosteroid produced naturally by the body, in the adrenal glands.

**cyanosis** A blue discoloration of the skin, lips and tongue resulting from the blood carrying too little oxygen. In asthma attacks it is a sign of a very serious condition, and requires emergency treatment with oxygen.

**dander** (also called 'animal dander') Contents of animal hair, or fur, which cause an allergic reaction.

**dehydration** A condition in which the body is deficient in water. In asthma, this may occur over several hours, as a result of rapid breathing, vomiting, and difficulty in drinking usual amounts of fluid.

**desensitization** If you have a strong allergy to a single allergen, it may be possible to treat it with desensitization. This is a series of injections over several weeks. They contain gradually increasing strengths of the allergen. The theory is that the body can build up a gradual resistance in this way, and that this removes the allergy. In practice, desensitizing treatments are not very effective and potentially dangerous. They are used now only in certain circumstances in specialist centres, for example for people with severe bee sting allergy.

**diurnal variation** A change from one time of day to another 12 hours later, usually from early hours of the morning to evening. In this book we talk mainly about diurnal variation in peak flow readings, and this means the difference between readings taken first thing in the morning (which tend to be lower), and those taken in the evening (which tend to be higher).

**dry powder devices** Inhalers in which the drug is delivered in the form of a powder, rather than an aerosol spray. The main types of dry powder devices are the Acuhaler (Figure 4.4), Aerolizer (Figure 4.5), Diskhaler (Figure 4.6), Easyhaler (Figure 4.7), Clickhaler (Figure 4.8), Novolizer (Figure 4.9), Pulvinal (Figure 4.10), Turbohaler (Figures 4.11 and 4.12) and Twisthaler (Figure 4.13).

**early onset asthma** Asthma that starts in childhood.

**eczema** (also called atopic eczema) This is a red, itchy inflammation of the skin, sometimes with blisters and weeping. There are several different types. Atopic eczema is common in children and is associated with other allergic conditions, particularly hay fever, and asthma.

**exercise-induced asthma** Symptoms of asthma brought on after several minutes of exercise, particularly running. Exercise is one of the most important triggers of asthma symptoms.

**extrinsic asthma** Asthma that is clearly triggered by some external factor, particularly allergens such as house dust mite and animal hair. The term 'atopic asthma' is used in preference nowadays.

**generic names** A general, or true, name for a medicine. Different from the brand name, which is given by the company that produces it. Any one drug can have several brand names but only one generic name.

**genes** A unit of heredity, which helps to make up an individual's characteristics. Genes are contained on chromosomes in all the cells of the body. Each individual has his or her own set of millions of genes – half of which are inherited from the mother and half from the father.

**hay fever** A condition of the nose and eyes caused by allergy to grass pollen during the summer months of June and July. Sometimes the same allergy also results in asthma symptoms – so-called 'pollen' asthma. Hay fever is also known as seasonal rhinitis.

**house dust mite** A microscopic insect, correct name *Dermatophagoides pteronyssinus*. It survives by feeding on the dead scales of human skin. We all shed these in great numbers, continuously, and they collect in house dust, particularly in bedding. The house dust mite is the most important and common cause of allergy and allergic asthma in the UK. Numbers are high all the year round, but especially so in the early winter months.

**hyperventilation** (also known as overbreathing) This is breathing more often than the body needs for its oxygen requirements and for getting rid of carbon dioxide. It occurs most often in periods of tension, anxiety or overexcitement.

**immune system** The body's own defences against outside
'attackers', whether they are infections, injuries or other agents
that are recognized as foreign, e.g. immunizations. The body's
immune system reacts by attacking them, and producing
antibodies, which give more long-lasting protection against future
attackers of the same type. For example, in an attack of measles,
the body's immune system fights off the infection after several
days, but also produces antibodies that will protect for many years
against a future attack.

**inflammation** The reaction of the body to some injury, infection or
disease process. Generally, its purpose is to protect the body against
the spread of injury or infection, but in some cases, as in asthma, the
inflammation becomes chronic, and this tends to damage the body
rather than protect it.

**intrinsic asthma** Asthma that is not obviously triggered by any
external agent, but tends to be continuous. The term 'non-atopic
asthma' is used in preference nowadays.

**late-onset asthma** Asthma that begins in adult life, with no past
history of it being a problem during childhood. Many people who
appear to have late-onset asthma will give a history of being 'chesty'
children, or having repeated 'bronchitis' or 'pneumonia' as children.
This suggests that their asthma is recurring in adulthood, rather than
appearing for the first time.

**late reaction** When people with asthma are exposed to triggers for
their asthma, they may react within minutes with symptoms. This is
usually easy to identify. However, there may be another 'late'
reaction, which occurs approximately 6–10 hours afterwards. This is
caused by a different set of reactions, but is every bit as important
as the short-term reaction. Because of the time gap, it is more
difficult to identify. It does not respond so well to reliever treatment
as the short-term reaction.

**leukotriene receptor antagonists (LTRAs)** LTRAs block one of
the inflammatory pathways in the airways that cause asthma
symptoms. They may be helpful in exercise-induced symptoms and
allergic rhinitis if asthma is present. They are a tablet medicine, not
an inhaler. They are used as **additional** treatment for asthma where
people do not improve with steroid preventers.

**litres per minute** The reading on the peak flow meter is measured in
litres per minute. It refers to the number of litres per minute that

would be blown out of the lungs if someone could continue blowing at their peak flow rate.

**long-acting relievers** These are two long-acting inhaled broncho-dilator drugs: salmeterol (Serevent) and formoterol (Oxis or Aerolizer). They are used in addition to inhaled steroids when asthma symptoms persist. They need be taken only twice daily.

**lungs** The organs of breathing. The function of the lungs is to take oxygen into the bloodstream, and to get rid of the waste product, carbon dioxide, into the exhaled air.

**medical history** Someone's past record of illnesses, symptoms and medical problems.

**monilia infection** Another name for **thrush** or infection with candida.

**morning dip** We all have a natural variation in our peak flow readings during day and night, which results in slightly lower readings in the morning than the evening. In asthma in general, and some people with asthma in particular, this pattern is very much exaggerated, so that a normal reading in the evening is followed by a pronounced 'dip' in the readings the following morning. This is recognized as an indication for changing treatment.

**nasal polyp** see **polyp**.

**NSAIDs** (full name non-steroidal anti-inflammatory drugs) A class of drugs used extremely commonly for arthritis, other rheumatic conditions and generally for pain relief. Brufen, Nurofen, Froben, Ponstan, ibuprofen, indomethacin, Feldene and Voltarol are well-known examples. All are related to aspirin, and in a few people can make asthma worse. They can also cause water retention, which may be a particular problem for people with heart or kidney disease.

**occupational asthma** Asthma that results purely as a consequence of working in a particular environment. Important examples are given in the section on *Work* in Chapter 6. Proven occupational asthma is a prescribed disease, meaning that industrial compensation may be available if cause and effect can be proved.

**oral steroids** Corticosteroid treatment given by mouth. Nearly always this is given as prednisolone tablets.

**osteoporosis** Thinning of the bones, which occurs as a result of overall loss of calcium from the body. The most important group affected by this is older women, who lose bone density more rapidly after their menopause. The results of osteoporosis are an increased risk of fractures, particularly of the spine and thigh bone.

**overbreathing** Another name for **hyperventilation**.

**ozone** A gas, related to oxygen, which is present in small amounts in the atmosphere.

**passive smoking** Breathing in smoke from another person's cigarette, cigar or pipe.

**peak expiratory flow (PEF)** In this book we also refer to peak flow rates, readings, charts, diaries, meters and monitoring! A PEF is a very simple but effective measure of how hard someone can blow air out of their lungs. The instrument used to measure it is a peak flow meter. If the airways are wide open then air can be blown out at a very high rate of litres per minute. If, as in asthma, the airways are narrowed down, then the PEF falls simply because air cannot be blown out at the same speed. A PEF reading is the measurement achieved on the scale of the meter; a peak flow chart is a record of PEF readings kept over a period of time, and a peak flow diary does the same, usually recording peak flow readings at particular times of day, and also keeping track of symptoms and treatment over the same time. Peak flow monitoring is usually carried out by the person with asthma. They have a home peak flow meter (available on National Health Service prescription) and can track their own condition, with assistance from their doctor or asthma nurse.

**photochemical smog** A very unhealthy atmosphere caused by a reaction between pollution near ground level and sunlight. This usually occurs in hot climates, where an urban environment is surrounded by mountains, which tend to trap the air, e.g. in places such as Los Angeles and Athens. It has occurred in the UK, especially in London. The smog contains gases that are damaging to the lungs, and can make asthma very much worse. These include ozone, particulate matter and oxides of nitrogen.

**placebo** A medicine that is inactive or ineffective. In clinical trials new drugs are tested against a placebo.

**pleura** Two layers of membrane surrounding and covering the lungs internally as a protection. Infection of the pleura results in pleurisy – a very painful condition.

**polyp** A small harmless growth, which arises from an internal lining of part of the body, such as the lining of the bowel, or the nose. Polyps in the nose are quite common in adults with asthma, particularly those whose asthma started later in life. (People with polyps may be allergic to aspirin.)

**preventers** Medicines that are taken to prevent the symptoms of asthma from occurring, rather than to relieve them when they do occur. The most important group of preventers is the inhaled steroid drugs, described in Chapter 4.

**prodromal** (as in prodromal itching) Symptoms coming before the start of an illness or a condition.

**propellants** These include CFCs (chlorofluorocarbons), which are now banned because of their effect on the environment, and HFAs (hydrofluoroalkanes), which have been developed to replace them.

**protectors** A term previously used to describe the first **long-acting reliever**.

**puffer** A popular name for a metered dose inhaler (MDI – Figure 4.1). The most commonly used inhalers release a puff of spray containing the drug when the canister is pressed.

**relievers** The most frequently used type of anti-asthma drug. Relievers relax muscle spasm (tightness) around the airways, helping to open up the airways and relieve symptoms. Relievers are best used when needed rather than regularly. The most frequently prescribed reliever inhalers are Ventolin (salbutamol) and Bricanyl (terbutaline). Reliever tablets and syrups – Bambec, Phyllocontin, Uniphyllin, Ventolin and Volmax – are sometimes prescribed. See also **long-acting relievers**.

**remission** A period of time without symptoms or problems from a condition. In asthma the most likely time for a remission to occur is in late childhood. The condition may go into remission for many years, and treatment will not be required during this time. Asthma is such an unpredictable condition that it may go into remission at any time. However, the opposite also applies – after remission it may return at any time.

**Reye's syndrome** Reye's syndrome is a rare condition almost always preceded by a viral infection, predominantly affecting children between 4 and 16 years. The use of salicylates, like aspirin, during viral disease appears to be statistically linked to the incidence of Reye's syndrome, even though there is no conclusive proof. Therefore parents are advised not to give children under 16 aspirin for viral infections.

**rhinitis** Inflammation of the lining of the nose – similar to the process of asthma in the airways. In the UK the most common reason for rhinitis is allergy to grass pollen (hay fever or seasonal rhinitis).

The symptoms of rhinitis are running of the nose, blocking, sneezing and itching.

**rhinovirus**  A type of virus known to cause the common cold frequently, and in people with asthma to provoke episodes of asthma with a cold (a 'cold going to the chest'), especially during the autumn and early winter months.

**season ticket**  Three-monthly or yearly prescription season tickets (prepayment) are available. Pharmacies, Post Offices, Benefits Agency offices or your doctor's surgery will have application forms. Alternatively they can be completed on line from the Prescription Pricing Authority (see *Appendix*).

**silent chest**  When someone is having a severe asthma attack, they have difficulty breathing air in and out of the chest. Usually, during an asthma attack, the person has very noisy, wheezy breathing that can be heard with a stethoscope. During a severe asthma attack very little air is moving through the air passages. If the doctor or asthma nurse tries to listens to the breath sounds with a stethoscope during this severe attack, they may not hear anything – hence the name 'silent chest'.

**skin prick tests**  Special tests to show whether a person has a tendency to allergy. Drops of solution containing allergen are placed on the forearm and the skin is pricked gently through the solution. A positive test occurs when a wheal, like a nettle rash, appears within 10 minutes. The tests are painless and inexpensive. The results of these tests may provide helpful information for the GP or nurse.

**spirometry**  This is a test for lung function using an instrument called a spirometer. It is sometimes used for asthma but more often to diagnose **chronic obstructive pulmonary disease** (COPD).

**steroids**  A particular group of chemicals that includes very important hormones, produced naturally by the body, and also many medicines used for a wide range of medical purposes. In asthma, the steroids with which we are concerned is the corticosteroids. Very often this term is shortened to steroids, causing people to confuse their asthma treatments with the anabolic steroids used for body building. Steroids provide two of the most important treatments for asthma: the tablet form (prednisolone), which is mainly used in short courses and can be a life saver in acute attacks; and the inhaled form which, as AeroBec, Becotide, Becloforte, Filair, Flixotide and

Pulmicort, comprises the most important type of preventive treatment.

**tartrazine** An additive, which formerly was found commonly in foods and soft drinks, but which is increasingly being removed. It is probably the most important food additive implicated in asthma.

**theophylline** Generic name for one of the reliever type of drugs. Theophylline can be taken by mouth, or given by injection. There is no inhaled form. They are used less often nowadays.

**thrush** (also called candida, monilia) A fungal infection of warm moist places in the body, particularly the mouth and skin folds. In asthma, thrush is an important side effect of inhaled corticosteroid treatment. It is also a frequent consequence of a course of antibiotic treatment. Usually it is easily treatable.

**topical (inhaled) steroids** Steroids that are inhaled or breathed in and so do not get absorbed directly into the bloodstream. This is an advantage, because it minimizes the risk of side effects. Inhaled topical steroids are used mainly in asthma (in inhaler devices) and in allergic rhinitis (e.g. hay fever).

**trachea** The main windpipe, which begins at the level of the voice box, and goes into the top of the chest, where it divides into the bronchi (**airways**).

**triggers** Factors that **may** bring on symptoms or attacks of asthma. They do not cause asthma. Examples are given in the section on *Triggers* in Chapter 2.

**twitchy airways** Another name for bronchial hyperreactivity.

**uncontrolled asthma** The most important stage of asthma for you to recognize! This is when asthma begins to deteriorate, and head towards an acute attack. If you can recognize it early, and take the right action, trouble will be avoided.

**upper respiratory tract infection (URTI)** An infection of the ears, nose and throat. The best known example is the common cold. Almost all URTIs are caused by viruses. This means they take their own time to disappear, and they are rarely helped by giving antibiotics, which do not have any effect on virus infections.

**virus** A microscopic organism, which multiplies in and attacks living cells, causing infections. There are many different groups of viruses and many thousands of different types of virus. The infections they cause vary enormously, from the trivial type to the fatal. Well-known examples are the common cold, influenza, measles, hepatitis and

AIDS. Virus infections are important in asthma because they are the commonest trigger for attacks. Colds going on to the chest, particularly in winter, are the triggers for many attacks. Virus infections are not helped by antibiotics.

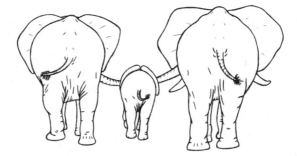

# Appendix
# Useful addresses, information and websites

## General

**Asthma UK**
(formerly known as the
**National Asthma Campaign**)
Summit House
70 Wilson Street
London EC2A 2DB
Tel: 020 7786 5000
Fax: 020 7256 6075
Asthma UK Adviceline (asthma
nurse specialists): 08457 01 02 03
Website: asthma.org.uk/adviceline
*Asthma UK produces excellent
information, including:*

- *action plans and a schools
  information pack (they have
  developed a school asthma
  policy document)*
- *insurance: Asthma UK will
  provide information and
  contact details if you are
  having problems obtaining
  travel insurance cover because
  of your asthma*
- *booklets and factfiles on any
  aspect of asthma*

- *frequently asked questions in a
  number of different languages*
- *a quarterly magazine for
  members called the* Asthma
  Magazine

**British Lung Foundation**
73–75 Goswell Road,
London EC1V 7ER
Tel: 020 7688 5555
Fax: 020 7688 5556
Helpline: 08458 50 50 20
(Mon–Fri 10 am–6 pm)
Website: www.lunguk.org
*BLF has a network of support
groups throughout the UK called
Breathe Easy. The website has
all the contact details for these
groups. Also produces excellent
booklets and information sheets.
The BLF has also set up Baby
Breathe Easy support groups
across the country. They produce
excellent booklets, information
sheets and a quarterly magazine
called* Breathing Space.

## Chest, Heart and Stroke Organisations

*Scotland*
65 North Castle Street
Edinburgh EH2 3LT
Tel: 0131 225 6963
Fax: 0131 220 6313
Advice line: 0845 077 6000
Website: www.chss.org.uk

*Northern Ireland*
22 Great Victoria Street
Belfast BT2 7LX
Tel: +44 (0)28 9032 0184
Fax: +44 (0)28 9033 3487
Helpline: 0845 769 7299
Website:
www.nichsa.com/html/index.php

## Mark Levy's website
Website: www.consultmarklevy.com

## National Health Service
The Department of Health
Website is available at:
www.dh.gov.uk

## National Institute for Health and Clinical Excellence (NICE)
Website: www.NICE.org.uk
*Produces guidelines for health professionals on the use of inhaler devices for children in both the under-5 and 5–15-year age groups.*

## Prescription Pricing Authority
Website: www.ppa.org.uk
*If you pay for your prescriptions it may be worthwhile buying a Prepayment Certificate for either 3 months or 1 year. The application form can be completed on-line.*

## The Royal National Institute for the Blind
Website: onlineshop.rnib.org.uk/
*The RNIB sells different coloured raised labels called 'Bumpons', which you could attach to inhalers to help identify them more easily.*

## Alerting systems

## MedicAlert
1 Bridge Wharf
156 Caledonian Road
London N1 9UU
Freephone: 0800 581420
Tel: 020 7833 3034
Fax: 020 7278 0647
Website: www.medicalert.org.uk
*MedicAlert provides a life-saving identification system for people with allergies and other medical conditions. This information can be very useful and in some situations life saving, where immediate information may be needed about your allergies. There is a small yearly charge to keep your details on the database and these should be updated as necessary.*

## Allergy

**Allergy UK**
3 White Oak Square
London Road
Swanley BR8 7AG
Helpline: 01322 619898
Website: www.allergyuk.org

- *Educational material for adults, teenagers and children*
- *Information on vacuum cleaners with HEPA (high-efficiency particulate arrest) filters, which trap small particles of dust. They are more expensive and scientific evidence of benefit is limited*

## Anaphylaxis

**Anaphylaxis Campaign**
PO Box 275
Farnborough GU14 6SX
Help Line: 01252 542029
Tel: 01252 373793
Fax: 01252 377140
Website:
www.anaphylaxis.org.uk/home.html

## Biomass fuels

Article on the BBC News website:
'UK boost for biomass fuel crops':
news.bbc.co.uk/1/hi/sci/tech/3746554.stm
(See Chapter 2.)

## Children and schools

**Department of Education and Skills/Department of Health**
Their publication *Managing medicines in schools and early years settings* (2005)
(Reference:1448-2005DCL-EN)
can be downloaded from
www.teachernet.gov.uk/publications.
Website:
www.teachernet.gov.uk/wholeschool/healthandsafety/medical/

## Eczema

**National Eczema Society**
Hill House, Highgate Hill
London N19 5NA
Tel: 020 7281 3553
Fax: 020 7281 6395
Eczema Help Line: 0870 241 3604
Website: www.eczema.org
*The National Eczema Society is a designated charitable organization specifically for people with eczema and they can provide practical help and information and support.*

## Education

**Boots the Chemist**
Website:
bootslearningstore.com/lunglab/teachers/
*Contains information on the lungs and asthma linked to the national educational curriculum.*

## Flying

The article here provides information and a summary of national recommendations for 'fitness to fly':
www.brit-thoracic.org.uk/docs/
   flyingguidelines.pdf

## Internet search engines

These are just a few of the more commonly used sites in the UK:

- Altavista: www.altavista.com
- Ask Jeeves: www.ask.com
- Google: www.Google.com
- Yahoo: www.yahoo.com

## Medicines

**British National Formulary**
Website: bnf.org/bnf
*For information on medicines.*

## Occupational asthma

**British Occupational Health Research Foundation (BOHRF)**
Websites:
www.bohrf.org.uk/content/asthma.htm
www.bohrf.org.uk/downloads/asthwork.pdf
*Produces guidelines for practice nurses and GPs to raise awareness of occupational asthma presenting in general practice. There is also an excellent guide on occupational asthma for employers, workers and their representatives.*

## Health and Safety Executive and the TUC

Website:
www.hse.gov.uk/asthma/index.htm
*Publishes a series of leaflets for people with asthma, employers and health professionals.*

## Pollen

**The National Pollen and Aerobiology Research Unit**
Website:
www.pollenuk.co.uk/aero/pm/PM2.html
*Based in Worcester, this unit provides information about pollen counts and pollen monitoring, useful for people with hay fever.*

## Smoking

Websites that give some help on giving up smoking:
www.givingupsmoking.co.uk/
www.dh.gov.uk/PolicyAndGuidance/Health
   AndSocialCareTopics/Tobacco/fs/en
www.ash.org.uk/html/factsheets/html/
   fact11.html

## Sports

**UK Sport**
Website: www.uksport.gov.uk/did/
*Useful drug information database where permitted or prohibited drugs can be identified for a wide range of sports.*

**World Anti-Doping Agency**
Website: www.wada-ama.org/
*Has very strict regulations on which drugs may be used in competitive sport.*

**Scuba diving**
Website:
www.brit-thoracic.org.uk/docs/diving.pdf
British Thoracic Society
Guidelines *for health professionals, on fitness for scuba diving.*

*Organizations for health professionals working with people with asthma*

**British Thoracic Society (BTS)**
Website: www.brit-thoracic.org.uk
*Current UK Asthma management guidelines are available on this site.*

**General Practice Airways Group (GPIAG)**
Website: www.gpiag.org
*A professional organization for primary carers with a specific interest in respiratory disease.*

**Scottish Intercollegiate Guideline Network (SIGN)**
Website: www.sign.ac.uk
*Current UK asthma management guidelines are available on this site.*

**Education for Health**
(incorporating National Respiratory Training Centre and Heartsave)
*A registered educational charity providing respiratory training programmes for health professionals. The courses are internationally recognized and there is a sister organization in the United States.*

*UK*
**Education for Health**
The Athenaeum
10 Church Street
Warwick CV34 4AB
Tel: 01926 838972
Fax: 01926 493224
Health Professional Helpline:
01926 493363
Website: www.educationforhealth.org.uk

*USA*
**National Respiratory Training Center**
711 W. North Street
Raleigh, NC 27603-1418
USA
Tel: +00 [1] 919-832-3539
Fax: +00 [1] 919-532-0382
Website: www.nrtc-usa.org/default.htm

*Manufacturers
of asthma medicines
and inhalers*

**Altana Pharma Ltd**
3 Globeside Business Park
Fieldhouse Lane
Marlow SL7 1HZ
Tel: 01628 646400
Fax: 01628 646443

• *Metered dose inhaler*

**AstraZeneca (UK) Ltd**
Horizon Place
600 Capability Green
Luton LU1 3LU
Medical Information Services:
Tel: 0800 783 0033
Fax: 01582 838003

• *Turbohaler*

• *Metered dose inhaler*

• *Nebuhaler*

• *Nebuchamber*

• *Accolate tablets*

**Boehringer Ingelheim**
Ellesfield Avenue
Bracknell RG12 8YS
Tel: 01344 424600
Fax: 01344 741738

• *Metered dose inhaler*

**Clement Clarke International**
Cartel Industrial Estate
Edinburgh Way
Harlow CM20 2TT
Tel: 01279 414969
Fax: 01279 635232

• *Mini-Wright Peak Flow Meter*

• *Able Spacer*

• *In-Check Dial*

**Ferraris Medical Ltd**
4 Harforde Court
John Tate Road
Hertford SG13 7NW
Tel: 01992 526300
Fax: 01992 526320

• *Ferraris Peak Flow Meter*

• *Pocket Chamber*

• *Piko (electronic peak flow
meter)*

**Fyne Dynamics Ltd**
1 Horsecroft Place
Pinnacles
Harlow CM19 5BT
Tel: 01279 423423
Fax: 01279 454373

• *Mag-Flo Inhaler Trainer*

• *MicroPeak Peak Flow Meter*

**GlaxoSmithKline**
Stockley Park West
Uxbridge UB11 1BT
Tel: 0800 221441
Fax: 0800 8900 4328

- *Metered dose inhaler*
- *Diskhaler*
- *Accuhaler*
- *Volumatic (withdrawn October 2005)*
- *Babyhaler*
- *Aerochamber spacer devices (sole distribution rights in UK)*

**Ivax Pharmaceuticals UK Ltd**
Ivax Quay, Albert Basin
Royal Docks
London E16 2QJ
Tel: 08705 020304
Fax: 08705 323334

- *Autohaler*
- *Easi-breathe*
- *Metered dose inhaler*

**3M Health Care Ltd**
3M House
Morley Street
Loughborough LE11 1EP
Tel: 01509 611611
Fax: 01509 237288
Helpline: 01509 613028

- *Metered dose inhaler*
- *Autohaler*

**Medeva Pharma Limited**
Medeva House
Regent Park Kingston Road
Leatherhead KT22 7PQ
Tel: 01372 364000
Fax: 01372 364050

- *Clickhaler*

**Merck Sharp & Dohme Ltd (MSD)**
Hertford Road
Hoddesdon EN11 9BU
Tel: 01992 467272
Fax: 01992 451066

- *Montelukast tablets*

**Micro Medical Ltd**
PO Box 6
Rochester ME1 2AZ
Tel: 01634 893500
Fax: 01634 893600

- *MicroPeak Peak Flow Meter*

**Ranbaxy (UK) Ltd**
6th Floor, CP House
97–107 Uxbridge Road
Ealing
London W5 5TL
Tel: 020 8280 1600
Fax: 020 8280 1616

- *Easyhaler*

**Rhône-Poulenc Rorer**
RPR House
50 Kings Hill Avenue
West Malling ME19 4AH
Tel: 01732 584000
Fax: 01732 584080

- *Spinhaler*
- *Metered dose inhaler*
- *Syncroner*

**Schering-Plough Ltd**
Unit 3 Shire Park
Falcon Way
Welwyn Garden City AL7 1TW
Tel: 01707 363636
Fax: 01707 363690

- *Twisthaler*

**Trinity-Chiesi
Pharmaceuticals**
Cheadle Royal Business Park
Highfield
Cheadle SK8 3GY
Tel: 0161 488 5555
Fax: 0161 488 5565

- *Pulvinal*

**Trudell Medical International**
Biocity Nottingham
Pennyfoot Street
Nottingham NG1 1GF
Tel: 0115 912 4380
Fax: 0115 912 4289

- *Aerochamber manufacturer*

**Viatris Pharmaceuticals Ltd**
Building 2000, Beach Drive
Cambridge Research Park
Waterbeach
Cambridge CB5 9PD
Tel: 01223 205999
Fax: 01223 205998

- *Novolizer*

**Vitalograph Ltd**
Maids Moreton
Buckingham MK18 1SW
Tel: 01280 827110
Fax: 01280 823302

- *Vitalograph Peak Flow Meter*

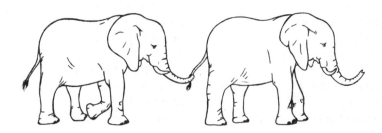

# Index

Page numbers in *italic* refer to illustrations. Those followed by italic *g* refer to the glossary.

Able Spacer 104, *108*, 116
   high doses of drug 120, 121, 144
   when breastfeeding 190
acaricide sprays 74
Accuhaler 89, *97*
acid in stomach 175
action plans *see* asthma action plans
acupuncture 77
acute 282*g*
acute asthma 25, 115
addiction, treatment not addictive 114
addresses 295–302
adhesives 195
adolescents 123, 225–6, 229, 246–7
   bone age 246
   *see also* puberty
adrenal glands 118–19, 282*g*
adrenaline 76, 261
   in competitive sports 209

AeroBec 80, 83, 91, 115
Aerochamber 104, *107*, *109*, 116
   high doses of drug 120, 121, 144
   when breastfeeding 190
Aerolin, when to take 91
Aerolizer *98*, 99
aerosol sprays 210
age
   continuing with treatment 163
   worsening of symptoms 219–20
   *see also* children; elderly people
air conditioning 193
air pollution 35, 65, 66, 193
   and weather 209–12
   *see also* atmospheric conditions
air purifiers 69
air quality, poor 196, 210–11
Airomir 80, 95, 141, 144, 145, 236
   in competitive sports 208
   when to take 91
airways *9*, 9–10, 282*g*
   inflammation/swelling of airway lining *10*, 11, 25, 66, 82, 84

airways ( *continued*)
  muscle contraction *10*, 11, 25,
    79
  narrowing *10*, 10, 11, 25, 51–2,
    64
  twitchy *see* twitchy airways
alcohol 192, 212–13
aldehydes 195, 213
allergens 12, 20, 28, 177, 282*g*
  allergen avoidance 69–75
allergic asthma 35, 59, 61
allergic reaction 282*g*
allergic rhinitis 28–9, 87, 177
allergies 12, 13, 28, 61, 176, 282*g*
  *v.* asthma 43, 62–3
  and home conditions 172
  skin prick test 35, 63–4, 73, 136,
    238, 292*g*
  as triggers 29
  very severe 260
  *see also* triggers; *and specific*
    *allergies*
Allergy UK 275, 297
alternative therapies *see*
    complementary therapies
altitude problems 198, 201, 202–3
altitude sickness 202, 267
aluminium 195
alveoli *9*, 9, 26, 66, 282*g*
Alvesco 80, 83, 117, 120, 145, 166,
    188
  when to take 91, 115
ambulance 256, 262
Ambulance Service as
    employment 197
aminophyllines 121, 238, 283*g*
ammonium chloride 195
anabolic steroids 115, 209, 283*g*
anaemia 90

anaesthetics 178–9
Anapen 261
anaphylactic attacks 185, 214, 215
anaphylaxis 283*g*
Anaphylaxis Campaign 275, 297
angina 221
animal dander (fur or hair) 28, 35,
    62, 71, 176, 286*g*
animals 29
  in workplace 193, 195
antibiotics 12, 90–1, 121
  allergies to 47
  manufacture 195
antibodies 16, 136, 181
anticholinergic drugs 113
antihistamine 261
anti-immunoglobulin E (IgE)
    125–6
anti-inflammatory drugs 80, 83,
    90, 283*g*
Armed Forces 197
aromatherapy 78
Asmabec 91, 115
Asmanex 80, 83, 87, 145, 166, 188
  high doses 120
  when to take 91, 115
Asmasal 80, 91
Asmasal Clickhaler *see* Clickhaler
aspirin 33–4, 61, 187, 220
asthma
  cardiac *v.* bronchial 10
  causes of 136–7
  chronic severe *see* brittle
    asthma
  how to beat 4
  long-term outlook 219–22
  not infectious 15
  related conditions 42–3, 61–2
  types of 12–15, 59–60

variability in severity of 8, 14–15
what it is 8–12, 64–5
asthma action plans 128–9, 131, 166–8
  **in emergency** 265
  for holidays 161
  written 157–61
asthma attacks
  acute 25, 40, 115
  care of someone with attack 262
  check-ups 259–60, 266, 271
  feeling strangled or suffocated 26
  no medication available 261–3
  prevention 143
  review after severe attack 132
  symptoms not improving 253
  unpredictability 40, 41, 142–3
  in winter 37
  *see also* **emergencies**
asthma clinics 131–40
asthma register 133, 283*g*
asthma review 126, 270–2, 279–80
Asthma UK 194, 201, 254, 274, 274–5, 295
  advice line 275, 277
  asthma in schools 240, 243
  leaflets 204, 266, *270–1*, 275, 276, *280*
  school information packs 240, 243, 281
  website 276
athletes 64
  athlete's passport 208
  *see also* sports
atmospheric conditions 211
  *see also* air pollution

atopic asthma 35
atopic eczema 27, 64, 191, 283*g*
atopy 20, 21, 42–3, 63–4, 238, 283*g*
atropine 76
Atrovent 113
Autohaler *95–7*, 95–7, *96*, 236

babies *see* infants
bakers 195
Beclazone, during pregnancy 188
Becloforte 83, 91, 123
beclometasone 83, 87, 117, 123, 166
  in competitive sports 209
  high doses 120
  inhalers 104, 145
  when to take 91
Beconase, *v.* Becotide 86–7
Becotide 80, 83, 123, 145, 163, 166
  *v.* Beconase 86–7
  in competitive sports 208–9
  effect on osteoporosis 118
  high doses 120
  during pregnancy 188
  *v.* Ventolin 84–5
  when breastfeeding 190
  when to take 91, 115
bee sting allergy 72
bereavement 41
beta-agonists (beta-stimulants) 89, 94, 283–4*g*
beta-blockers 34, 94, 220–1, 284*g*
BHR *see* bronchial hyperreactivity
biomass fuels 37, 297
birds 29
blood, giving 178
blood pressure, high 34, 43, 116
blood tests 64, 73, 121, 238

blue discoloration *see* cyanosis
body hair, overgrowth of 90
bone age 246, 284*g*
bone densitometry 192
bones
  promoting healthy 192
  thinning of *see* osteoporosis
booklets *see* information on
    asthma
bottle-feeding 21
Braille labels for devices 277–8
brand names of drugs 80, 217–18,
    284*g*
breastfeeding 20, 21, 190–1
breath, shortness of 11, 24, 25, 31
breath-activated devices 284*g*
  for child's use away from home
    235
  inhalers 89, *95–7*
Breathe Easy 276, 295
breathing
  during childbirth 189–90
  controlled 79
  exercises 77–8, 79, 239
  into paper bag 264–5
  slowly and regularly 258,
    264–5
  and swimming 205
  *see also* breathlessness;
    hyperventilation; wheezing
breathlessness 40
  **in emergency** 253, 256, 258,
    265
Bricanyl 89, 112, 145, 178
  in competitive sports 208
  **emergency situations** 255,
    262
    away from home 161, 204
  before exercise 206

increasing need for 114, 141–2
not working 255
*v.* Pulmicort 83, 88
side effects 113
when to take 82, 85, 91, 115
British Lung Foundation 274, 275,
    276, 295
  booklets 276
British National Formulary 298
British Occupational Health
    Research Foundation 194,
    298
British Thoracic Society (BTS)
    279, 299
brittle asthma 17, 252, 259, 284*g*
bronchi *9*, 9–10, 284*g*
bronchial asthma 10
bronchial hyperreactivity (BHR)
    15–16, 20, 32, 284–5*g*
  *see also* twitchy airways
bronchioles *9*, 9, 26, 284*g*
bronchiolitis 232, 285*g*
bronchitis 65, 220, 222, 285*g*
bronchodilators 84, 89, 91, 206,
    285*g*
bruising of skin 116
budesonide 81, 83, 87, 145, 166,
    267
  high doses 120
  when to take 91
Bumpons 278
Buteyko 77

cabinet makers 195
caffeine, in competitive sports
    209
calcium 192
calcium loss in body 118
calorie needs in children 239

Candida infection *see* thrush
carbon dioxide 8, 9
cardiac asthma 10, 65, 285*g*
cards, warning (to show doctors) 119
carpets 70–1, 74
carrying heavy weights 172–3
cats 12, 28, 29, 38–9, 61, 62, 71–2, 180–1, 228, 238
causes of asthma 136–7
    *v.* triggers 29–30
central heating 37, 176–7, 193
CFCs *see* chlorofluorocarbons
charities for people with asthma 274
    sponsored events 275
check-ups 259–60, 266, 271
Chest, Heart and Stroke Association 275, 276, 296
chest pain 27–8
chest tightness 24, 25, 35, 221, 226, 255–6
childhood asthma 14, 17–18
children
    ability to control their own treatment 234–6
    affected by steroids 117, 120, 122–3
    altering medication 164–5, 166–7
    aspirin and 33–4
    benefits of sport 206–7
    blowing tests 60
    bone age 246, 284*g*
    breathlessness 143–4, 265
    calorie needs 239
    chances of developing asthma 41
    chest tightness 226

cystic fibrosis 65
deaths from asthma 17, 260–1
diagnosing asthma in 225, 226–7, 239
**emergency hospital admission** 250, 258–9
family history of allergies 227, 228
fear of overdosing 237–8
food allergy 17
gender and development of asthma 225–6, 229
'growing out of' asthma 219–20, 220, 225, 244–5
growth in 236–7
holiday precautions 203–4
hygiene hypothesis 19, 181
hyperactivity 123
inhaled steroids 117, 122–3
judging severity of asthma 230
late maturity 246
medical history 226
occurrence of asthma 225–6
peak flow meter/tests *150*, 155, 227
physical/emotional maturity 246
playing with devices 244
pulse rate 265
skin prick tests 238
smoking by parents/family 172, 182–3, 227, 228
sweat test 65
syrup form of reliever 122
treatment not addictive 114
vomiting 234
weight loss 239
wheezing 60
*see also* adolescents; infants; puberty; school

Chinese medicine 76
chlorine 205
chlorofluorocarbons (CFCs) 104, 210
chrome 195
chronic 285*g*
chronic bronchitis 65, 220, 222
chronic obstructive pulmonary disease (COPD) 62, 65, 285*g*
ciclesonide 83, 117, 120, 145, 166, 188
ciclosporin 90
cigarettes *see* smoking
cimetidine 121, 195
circadian rhythm 175
claustrophobia 42
Clickhaler *100*, 101, 200, 236
climate *see* weather
coal burning 209
cobalt 195
codeine 231
coffee beans 195
cold air, as trigger 32, 35, 37, 176, 177, 201, 202
cold cures, in competitive sports 209
colds 12, 14, 15, 18, 27, 29, 37, 38, 46, 47
    in children 30, 226, 228, 244
    continuing higher dose of inhaler 267–9
colophony 195
colour blindness 278
combination treatments 81
communication between doctor and patient 139–40
complementary therapies 75–9, 285–6*g*
    *see also individual therapies*

condoms 185
confidentiality 133–4
constipation 113
contraceptive pill 186, 187–8
control of asthma 38, 43, 88, 118
    and growth 236–7, 239
    long-term outlook 219–22
    patient involvement in 129–30
    *see also* PEF (peak expiratory flow); uncontrolled asthma
COPD *see* chronic obstructive pulmonary disease
corticosteroids 88, 115, 116, 286*g*
    in competitive sports 208
cortisol 119, 286*g*
cortisone 175, 286*g*
cost of treatments 8, 171–2, 218
cough medicines 177–8, 231
coughing 11, 24, 25, 27, 33, 35, 47
    in children 226, 231
    cold weather 32
    only at night 84
    tickly, as warning of attack 252
courses for health professionals 254
croup 231
cure for asthma 16
Customs 203
cyanosis (blue discoloration) 26, 252, 265, 286*g*
cystic fibrosis 65

dander *see* animal dander
dangers of drug treatments 121
Datura 76
death 16–17, 17, 260–1
dehydration 267, 286*g*
Department of Education and Skills 297

Department of Health 297
depression 40–1
    postnatal 41
desensitization treatment 72, 286*g*
detergent manufacturing 195
devices 94–111
    *see also* dry powder devices;
        spacer devices; *and specific*
        *devices*
diabetes 43, 116
diagnosis of asthma 46–50, 58–9
    hair analysis and iridology 78
    importance of early diagnosis
        225, 239
    tests 50–8
diary chart
    for peak expiratory flow 53,
        173, 187, 194
    for symptoms 48, *49*
diclofenac 33
diesel fumes 209
diet 129–30, 192
    exclusion diets 213–14
    *see also* alcohol; food allergy
Diskhaler 89, *98*, 99, 235
diurnal variation 286*g*
doctors *see* general practitioners;
        medical advice
dogs 28, 29, 35, 38–9, 61, 175–6
dosage of drugs *see* drugs, dosage
drink *see* alcohol
drug manufacture 195
drugs 79–94
    allergies to 47, 61
    brand names 80, 217–18, 284*g*
    confiscation of 203
    dosage
        fear of overdosing 237–8,
            243, 262

higher dose after colds 267–9
    increasing 85, 160, 162
    reducing 164–5
    reducing and discontinuing
        163
    repeating 260
generic names 80, 217–18, 287*g*
immunosuppressive 90
keep taking 130
making asthma worse 33–4
not addictive 114
placebos 78
during pregnancy 189
stopping completely 166
therapeutic use exemption
    (TUE) for sport 208
*see also* side effects; treatment;
    *and individual drugs and*
    *drug groups*
dry powder devices 89, 97–104,
    286–7*g*
    for child's use 235–6, 244
    effect on teeth 123
    may be affected by humidity
        and temperature 200
dust 43, 65, 175, 175–6, 176, 196
    as trigger 51, 228
    wood dusts 36, 195
    in workplace 193
dyes 195

E numbers (food additives) 215
early-onset asthma 13
Easi-breathe 95–7, *96*, 236
Easyhaler *99*, 99, 236
eczema 42, 47, 61, 287*g*
    and asthma 92–3, 245
    atopic 27, 64, 191, 283*g*
    connection with asthma 64

eczema (*continued*)
    in family history 228
education 297
Education for Health 254, 256,
        299
eggs 213
elderly people
    chronic obstructive pulmonary
        disease 62, 65
    need to be on oxygen 222
    osteoporosis 118
    pneumonia 92
    tuberculosis and asthma 66–7
    worsening of symptoms
        219–20
electrocardiogram (ECG) 221
**emergencies** 26
    advice after severe attack 132
    children on school trips 204
    drugs not working or effects
        not lasting 82, 84, 114, 142
    first aid for 253–4, 255
    making a spacer device 144,
        262, *263*
    medical care abroad 198
    panic and breathlessness
        143–4
    PEF problem on holiday 161
    silent chest 254
    treatment on certain airlines
        200
    warning signs of attack 250,
        251–3
        action to take 255–65
**emergency asthma packs** 199
emollients 87, 92–3
emotional factors 29, 31–2, 38,
        41–2
    *see also* depression; stress

emphysema 65, 66, 220, 222
employment *see* occupational
        asthma; work; workplace
energy, lack of 28
environmental factors 171
    as triggers 13, 16, 29
    *see also* smoking; social
        background; workplace
ephedra 76
ephedrine (adrenaline) 76
Epipen 261
episodic asthma 46
epoxy resin hardening agents 195
erythromycin 121
excitement, as trigger 29, 31–2, 38
exclusion diets 213–14
exercise 35, 38, 65, 129
    benefits of regular 204–5, 222
    breathing exercises 77–8, 79,
        239
    carrying heavy weights 172–3
    at high altitude 201
    and osteoporosis 118
    sports/PE at school 240, 241,
        243
    as trigger 13, 51, 172–3, 201,
        205–6, 228, 234
    walking 192
    weight-bearing 192
exercise-induced asthma 287*g*
exercise testing 59
exhaustion 265
Expert Patient Groups 276
extrinsic asthma 61, 287*g*
eye drops 94, 221
eyesight, poor 277–8

face, fullness ('moonface') 116
facemasks 104, *108–10*, 231, 232

farmers 195
feathers 28
Filair 80, 83
fire service 197
**first aid for emergencies** 253–4, 255
*see also* **emergencies**
fish 215
Flixonase 87
Flixotide 80, 81, 83, 87, 124–5, 145, 166
high doses 120
during pregnancy 188
when breastfeeding 190
when to take 91, 115
flour, as trigger 29, 195
'flu 92
fluid, in lungs 65
fluticasone 81, 83, 87, 120, 124–5, 145, 166
flying 199–200, 298
fog 211
follow-up appointments 133, 135
food allergy 17, 43, 47, 213–15
additives 215
**emergency kit** 260–1
exclusion diets 213–14
football 206–7, 208
Foradil 80, 89, 145, 156
side effects 113
when to take 91
forgetting to take inhalers 85
formoterol 80, 81, 89, 145, 267
side effects 113
when to take 91
fractures, tendency to 118, 191–2
fruit 215
fumes 29, 35, 59, 65, 176, 196, 209
from motor exhausts 209

in school science classes 240
in workplace 193
fungus infection 119

games *see* exercise; sports
gas burning 209
gas fires/cookers 37, 193, 210
gender, and asthma development 225–6, 229
General Practice Airways Group (GPIAG) 299
general practitioners (GPs)
consultation with 131–40
**emergency cover** 259
GMS contract 216
GP–patient relationship 139–40
questions to ask 4
generic names of drugs 80, 217–18, 287*g*
genes 18, 287*g*
genetic predisposition 229
Germany 209
glaucoma 34, 94, 221
GPs *see* general practitioners
grains 195
grass pollen 12, 28, 35, 62, 93–4, 177
'growing out of' asthma 219–20, 220, 225, 244–5
growth, steroid effect on 117, 122–3
growth hormone 175, 236–7
guided self-management 162
guidelines 279
guinea pigs 39

hair analysis 78
hamsters 39
hands, trembling 113

hardwoods 74, 195
hay fever 13, 27, 29, 46–7, 93, 287*g*
    associated with asthma 42, 61,
        245
    in family history 228
    homeopathy and 79
    inhaled steroid preventers 87
    and school exams 246–7
Health and Safety Executive 194,
        277, 298
health professionals,
        occupational risk 195
heart conditions 28, 34, 65, 221–2
heart failure 10, 65
Heartsave 254, 299
heel prick test 65
herbal remedies 76
heredity *see* inheritance
HFA (hydrofluoralkane)
        propellants 104
hoarseness of voice 116
holidays 198–204
    action plan 161
    children 203–4
    **emergencies** 161, 198
    health insurance 161, 198, 202
    keeping inhalers with you
        198–9, 199–200, 204
    oxygen shortage 198, 200
    review before going away 132,
        171
holistic approach to treatment 77
homeopathy 76, 77, 78–9
hormone replacement therapy
        (HRT) 118, 191
hormones 171, 175, 187–8
    growth hormone 175, 236–7
    as triggers 13, 29, 39
horses 28, 39, 48, 61

hospital care
    admissions 128, 250
    away from home 198, 261–2
    **emergency** 256, 258–9
    going straight to hospital 258–9
    'open door policy' 259
    *see also* anaesthetics; surgical
        operations
house dust mites 12, 28, 29, 35,
        37, 61, 62, 177, 287*g*
    in bedding 70, 72–4, 175
    and central heating 176
    getting rid of 69–70
    at high altitudes 202
    on soft toys 74
    as trigger 211
HRT (hormone replacement
        therapy) 118, 191
hydrofluoralkane (HFA)
        propellants 104
hygiene hypothesis 19, 181
hyperactivity in children 123
hyperventilation (overbreathing)
        77, 79, 144, 258, 264–5, 287*g*
hypnosis 77, 78

ibuprofen 33, 187
immune system 16, 19, 90, 120,
        172, 288*g*
immunizations, in children 230
immunotherapy 72
income support 217
Indian medicine 76
indigestion 88–9
indomethacin 33
industrial compensation 195
infants 225, 231–4
    breastfeeding as protection
        190–1

cough mixtures 231
croup 231
diagnosis 227
difficulty with facemask 231,
    232
heel prick tests 65
and parental smoking 172,
    182–3
risks before birth 188, 189
tests 227
treatment before asthma
    develops 232–3
see also adolescents; children;
    school
infection 13, 46, 121
see also viruses and viral
    infections; and individual
    infections
inflammation 288g
of airway lining 11, 66, 82, 84
influenza ('flu) 92
information on asthma 240, 243,
    276–80
Asthma UK leaflets 204, 266,
    270–1, 275, 276, 280
British Lung Foundation
    booklets 276
multilingual 275, 277
school information packs 240,
    243, 281
inhaled steroids see steroids,
    inhaled
inhalers
altitude affecting 201
availability abroad 200–1
blue 112, 123, 185, 241
breath-activated 89, 95–7, 284g
dependency on inhalers 115,
    243

before exercise 205–6
guidelines for children 279
higher dose after colds 267–9
how often to use 82–3
keeping them with you 145,
    199–200
on holiday 198–9, 199–200,
    204
in school 241, 241–2, 247
metered dose see metered dose
    inhalers
not addictive 114
spare 190, 201, 204, 247
use at room temperature 200
inheritance of asthma 15, 16,
    18–22, 47
injections 115, 125–6
not permitted in competitive
    sports 209
insects in workplace 195
insurance
health insurance on holiday
    161, 198, 202
life/sickness benefit 180
Intal 80, 83, 166
before exercise 206
International Olympic Committee
    (IOC) 208
Internet, search engines 298
intrinsic asthma 61, 288g
ionizers 69–70
ipratropium bromide 113
iridology 78
irritants, as triggers 13
isocyanates 195
isoprenaline 209
itching 27, 252, 254
prodromal 254, 291g

Japanese medicine 76
jobs *see* occupational asthma;
    work; workplace
Junifen 33

Kanpo 76
kidney damage 90

laboratory workers 195
lacquers, surface 195
lactose 123
lamb, in basic diet 214
larynx (voice box) 231
late-onset asthma 13, 21, 30,
    220–1, 288*g*
late reaction 35, 48, 288*g*
latex allergy 29, 185, 195
laughter as trigger 29, 31–2, 35,
    51
leaflets *see* information on
    asthma
learning points 4
leukotriene receptor antagonists
    81, 206, 237, 288*g*
Levy, Mark, website 296
lightheadedness 252, 264
linoleum floor covering 74
literature *see* information on
    asthma
long-term outlook 219–22
LTRAs *see* leukotriene receptor
    antagonists
lungs 8–10, *9*, 26, 289*g*
    breathing during childbirth 189
    fluid in 65
    growth in children 183
    lung function
        decreasing with age 220, 222
        improved with exercise 205

rhythm 175
scuba diving 207
strengthening 238–9
problems in women smokers
    182
scar tissue 65, 66

Ma Huang 76
management of asthma
    aim of 30–1, 82
    *see also* self-management
manufacturers 300–2
masks 104, *108–10*, 231, 232
mattresses 73–4
MDI *see* metered dose inhalers
meat tenderizing 195
MedicAlert 223, 296
medical advice
    asthma attack 270–1
    attack when no medication
        available 261–3
    away from home 198
    children 248
    **emergency situations** 251,
        261, 264, 265, 270–2
    giving blood 178
    how to seek 139–40
    judging severity of asthma in
        child 230
    monitoring symptoms 43
    occupational risks 196
    treatment for examination
        stress 247
    uncontrolled asthma 260, 266
    use of preventers in school 240
    *see also* asthma clinics; general
        practitioners; National
        Health Service; nurses' role
medical history 289*g*

medication/medicine *see* drugs;
    treatment
mefenamic acid 187
menopause 191–2
menstruation *see* periods
    (menstrual)
metals as risks 195
metered dose inhalers *94–5*, 104,
    291*g*
    children's use 235, 236, 244
    cleaning 140–1
    failure to work 140–1
    judging how full they are 141
methotrexate 90
milk, cow's 213–14, 215
    and breast milk 191
miners 65
Mini-Wright peak flow meter *146*,
    155, 277–8
moisturizing creams 87, 92–3
mometasone 83, 87, 120, 145, 166,
    188
monilia infection 289*g*
    *see also* thrush
montelukast 94, 189, 206, 237
mood changes 123
Moorhouse, Adrian 205
morning dip in PEF 53, 289*g*
mould spores 28, 176
mountain sickness 202, 267
mouth 91, 116–17, 119–20
mucus 11, 25, 59, 84, 266
multilingual advice 275, 277
muscles
    around airways *10*, 11, 25, 79
    heart 221–2
    increasing bulk 209
    between ribs 27
    trembling 113

Nasonex 87
National Asthma Campaign (now
    Asthma UK) 274
    *see also* Asthma UK
National Blood Service 178
National Eczema Society 297
National Health Service 171–2,
    216, 216–19, 296
    treatment away from home 261
National Institute for Health and
    Clinical Excellence (NICE)
    279, 296
National Pollen and Aerobiology
    Research Unit 298
National Respiratory Training
    Center, USA 299
National Respiratory Training
    Centre, UK *see* Education
    for Health
naturopathy 78
Nebuchamber 104, *106*, *110*, 111,
    116
    for high doses 120, 121, 144
Nebuhaler 104, *106*, *108*, 116
    for high doses 120, 121, 144
nebulizers 179, 264
nedocromil sodium 83, 166, 237
nervous problems and asthma
    40–1
New Zealand 209
nickel 195
night-time symptoms 24–5, 44, 47,
    89, 174–5
non-allergic asthma 59, 61
non-steroidal anti-inflammatory
    drugs (NSAIDS) 33–4, 187,
    220, 289*g*
nose
    itching as warning sign 252

nose (*continued*)
 nasal polyps 43, 61, 62, 87, 290*g*
 reaction to NSAIDS 33
Novolizer *100*, 101, 278
NSAIDS *see* non-steroidal anti-
 inflammatory drugs
Nuelin 121, 238
Nurofen 33, 187
nurses' role 131–3, 138–9
nut allergy 17
nuts 215

obstructive sleep apnoea 36
occupational asthma 13, 14, 29,
 30, 47, 59–60, 193–4, 289*g*
 guidelines 194
 information 277
 jobs/substances associated
 with 136–7, 195
occupational rhinitis 194
occupational therapy 65
occupational triggers 29
occupations *see* work; workplace
ointments 92–3
omalizumab 126
oral steroids 88, 116, 289*g*
osteoporosis 116, 117, 118, 121,
 191–2, 289*g*
overbreathing *see*
 hyperventilation
overdosing of drugs 237–8, 243
Oxis 80, 81, 89, 145, 156
 side effects 113
 when to take 91
oxygen 65
 in bloodstream 8, 9, 28, 221
 when flying 199
 and getting older 222
 given via cannula 222

shortage of
 in attacks 26, 221, 264, 267
 in emphysema 66
 during holidays/travel 198,
 202
ozone 210, 211, 290*g*

paints 195, 210
Pakistani medicine 76
palpitations 113, 221
panic and breathlessness 143–4
paracetamol 34
parents'/family smoking habits
 172, 182–3, 227, 228
passive smoking 33, 65, 171, 182,
 183–4, 290*g*
Patient Forum 219
peak expiratory flow *see* PEF
peanut allergy 213–14, 215, 260
pears, in basic diet 214
PEF (peak expiratory flow) 3,
 51–8, 290*g*
 action levels *158–9*, 158–9, 160,
 *269*
 action plans 157
 best readings 158–60
 calculating percentages 158–9
 charts *52–6*, *58*, *147*, *149–53*,
 163, 166–8, *167*, *173–4*,
 *268–9*
 asthma out of control *150*
 diurnal variation 151, 286–7*g*
 dropping below normal 160,
 252, 265, 268
 **emergency on holiday** 161
 guide to adjusting treatment,
 diary card record 173, 187,
 194, 215
 litres per minute 156, 288–9*g*

meters 3, 128, 145–6, *146*
  Braille labels for 277–8
  different readings between
    meters 156
  how to obtain one 154
  judging severity of episode
    230
  normal/best value reading
    145–8, *146*
  reasons for use 145–6
  usefulness of 128, 152–4
  variation in readings 53–5
  when to record 148–9
monitoring 145–56, 186–7
morning dip *153*, 154, 155, 252,
    289*g*
peak flow diary 53
preparation of 149–51
role in diagnosis 51–2, 57
variations in readings,
    calculating 165
warning of attack 153–4, 252
penicillin allergy 43, 47, 62
perfumes 210
periods (menstrual) 29, 39, 171,
    186–7
petrol fumes 209
pets 38–9, 71–2, 180–1
  *see also* cats; dogs
pharmacists 133
phlegm 11, 25, 84, 88, 91
photochemical smog 210, 290*g*
physiotherapy 65, 239
Pickering, Karen 204
pillows 72–3
placebos 78, 290*g*
planning *see* asthma action plans
platinum salts 195
pleura 27, 290*g*

pneumonia 92
Pocket Chamber 104, *107*, *109*,
    116
  for high doses 120, 121, 144
  when breastfeeding 190
police 197
pollen asthma 13–14
pollens 29, 43, 46, 211
  desensitizing treatment 72
  grass pollen 12, 28, 35, 62,
    93–4, 177
  during thunderstorms 211, 212
  tree pollen 28, 93–4
pollution, indoor 210
  *see also* air pollution
polyps *see* nose, nasal polyps
polyurethane manufacture 195
Ponstan 187
postnatal depression 41
practice nurse *see* nurses' role
prednisolone 88–9, 160
  children and 117, 144, 237
  dosage 88
  **in emergencies** 130, 161, 256
    away from home 204
    recorded on charts *149*, *152*
  side effects 88, 118–19, 120
pregnancy 29, 39–40, 171, 172,
    182, 188–91
  medication during 189
  prescription charges 217
  smoking during 16, 20
Prescription Pricing Authority 296
prescriptions
  charges 81–2, 92
  exemption from charges 217
  free in Wales 81
  generic prescribing 217–18
  for peak flow meter 154, 156

prescriptions (*continued*)
  repeat 130, 135
  season ticket 217, 292*g*
prevalence of asthma 8
preventers 32, 80, 83, 115, 199
  for the chest 87
  how often to use 84
  increasing dosage 85
  low dose inhaled steroids 122
  need for higher doses 141,
    160–1, 173–4, 267
  for the nose 87
  during pregnancy 188
  *v.* relievers 83, 84, 85–6, 115,
    141, 142
  taking on holiday 199
  treatment regularity 82, 83, 85,
    89, 91–2
  upper dose limit 237
  when to take 91–2
  *see also* steroids, inhaled
problem solving 4
prodromal itching 254, 291*g*
progesterone hormone therapy
  187
propellants (in inhalers) 104, 201,
  210, 291*g*
protectors 291*g*
  *see also* relievers, long-acting
proteolytic enzymes 195
psychological condition, asthma
  not 40
puberty 123, 244, 245
public houses 184–5
puffers 291*g*
  *see also* metered dose inhalers
Pulmicort 80, 81, 83, 87, 145, 166
  *v.* Bricanyl 83, 88
  high doses 120

  during pregnancy 188
  when to take 91, 115
pulmonary rehabilitation 65
pulse rate increase 235, 265
Pulvinal 83, *101*, 101–3, 200
Pulvinal beclometasone 91, 115,
  188
Pulvinal salbutamol 145, 236
  in competitive sports 208

Qvar 80, 83, 104, 115
  during pregnancy 188
  when to take 91

Radcliffe, Paula 204
rashes 27, 90
RAST blood test 64
reflexology 78
related conditions 42–3, 61–2
relaxation 79, 247, 258
relievers 32, 291*g*
  becoming reliant on them 115
  blue inhalers 112, 123, 185, 241
  bronchodilators 84, 89, 91, 206,
    285*g*
  **emergency situations** 84,
    161, 255, 260
  failure of repeated doses 260
  high doses 237
  increasing dosage 173–4
  keeping inhalers with you
    always *see under* inhalers
  long-acting 80–1, 289*g*
  not working or effects not
    lasting 84
  overdosing fears 237–8, 243,
    262
  *v.* preventers 83, 84, 85–6, 115,
    141, 142

short-acting 81
side effects 113
when to take 91–2
when unsuccessful 114
remission of symptoms 16, 163,
    291g
respiration 9
    see also breathing
respiratory symptoms 44, 46
reversibility of symptoms 64
reversibility testing 59
Reye's syndrome 34, 291g
rhinitis 30, 81, 94, 291–2g
    allergic 28–9, 87, 177
    occupational 194
    seasonal see hay fever
    vasomotor 177
Rhinocort 87
rhinoviruses 12, 292g
ribs 27
Royal National Institute for the
    Blind 278, 296

St John's Wort 76
Salamol 80, 145
salbutamol 80, 83, 112, 144, 145
    child's ability to judge dose
        234–6
    in competitive sports 208
    emergency situations 255,
        256
        away from home 161, 204
    increasing need for 141–2
    inhalers 104
    not working 255
    before sexual intercourse 185
    side effects 113
    in syrup form 122
    when to take 82, 91

saliva, animal 39
salmeterol 80, 81, 89, 145
    as extra treatment 156
    side effects 113
    when to take 91
sawdust 36
scar tissue in lungs 65, 66
Scholes, Paul 204
school 240–4
    holiday precautions 203–4
    information packs 240, 243, 281
    involving teacher 240, 242–3
    keeping inhalers with you 241,
        241–2, 247
    prevalence of asthma in 225
    school exams 246–7
    science classes 240
    sports and PE 240, 241, 243
    teachers' understanding 240,
        241–4
    see also adolescents; children;
        infants
Schools Asthma Policy Document
    243
Scottish Intercollegiate Guideline
    Network (SIGN) 279, 299
scuba diving 207, 299
self-help see self-management
self-management 273–81
    in emergency 265
    guided 162
    own responsibility in control of
        asthma 129–30
    see also asthma action plans
semen (sperm) allergy 185
Seretide 81
Serevent 80, 81, 89, 145
    as extra treatment 156
    side effects 113

Serevent (*continued*)
  when to take 91
sexual intercourse 185–6
shaking or trembling of hands 113
shellfish 215
shortness of breath 11, 24, 25, 31
sickness sensation 252, 264, 266
side effects of drugs 111–25
  growth in children 117, 122–3
  on immune system 120
  inhaled relievers 113
  inhaled steroids 116–17, 124
  one way of reducing 120
  osteoporosis 118, 121
  risk of increasing doses 121
  thrush of mouth or throat 91,
    116–17, 119, 120
  *see also under individual*
    *drugs*
silent chest 26, 254, 292*g*
Singulair 94, 237
skiing 201–2
skin
  rashes 27
  thinning/bruising of 116
  tingling or itching of 252, 254,
    264
skin conditions 43, 62, 214
skin prick tests 35, 63–4, 73, 136,
  292*g*
  children 238
skydiving 207
Slo-Phyllin 121, 238
smog, photochemical 210
smoking 21, 29, 44, 65, 66, 112,
  176, 181–5
  affecting heart 222
  breastfeeding and 190, 191
  and emphysema 66

and osteoporosis 118
by parents/family 172, 182–3,
  227, 228
passive 33, 65, 171, 182, 183–4,
  290*g*
during pregnancy 16, 20, 172
and social background 172
stopping 44, 60, 130, 183, 192,
  228–9
websites 298
women 181–2
in the workplace 183–4, 193,
  196
smoky environment 33, 184–5,
  193, 196, 210
  as trigger 46, 51, 60
sneezing 93
snoring 36
social background 172
sodium cromoglicate 83, 166, 206,
  237
sodium metabisulphate 215
soft/fizzy drinks 213, 215
soft furnishings 74
soldering 29, 59
soldering flux 195
spacer devices 104–11, 121, 144
  **emergency device,**
    **improvised** 144, 262, *263*
  **emergency treatment** 255,
    256, 257, *263*
  for higher doses of inhaled
    steroids 116–17, 120
  washing 110–11
  when breastfeeding 190
  *see also individual devices*
sperm allergy 185
spices 193
spirometry 51, 52–8, 227, 292*g*

sports 204–9
   avoidance of certain 207
   for children 206–7, 240, 241,
      243
   competitive sports and drugs
      208–9
   *see also* exercise; *and*
      *individual sports*
spots on throat 116, 119
sprays 196
stainless steel 195
stairs, climbing 31
statistics
   age of symptom development
      245
   atopy 63, 64
   cost to country of asthma 8,
      218
   deaths from asthma 16–17, 17,
      260
   hospital admissions 128, 250,
      258
   post-natal depression 41
   prevalence 8
   treatment of asthma during
      pregnancy 188
steroids 80, 93, 115–19, 292–3*g*
   anabolic 115, 283*g*
   cream 92–3
   dosage 87
   growth in children 117, 122–3
   high doses 121
   inhaled 83, 84–5, 293*g*
      children 117, 122–3
      high doses 116–17, 117, 120
      side effects 116–17, 124
      when to take 91
      *see also* preventers
   by injection 115
   long term 119
   low doses 116, 122
   oral 88, 116, 289*g*
   side effects 115–16
   stopping them after attack
      166–8
   tablets 115–16, 117, 118, 119,
      120, 261, 264
      **in emergencies** 256, 257
      osteoporosis and 191–2
      during pregnancy 40
   topical 293*g*
   *see also* corticosteroids; *and*
      *individual steroids*
stings 72
stomach ulceration 116
stomach upsets 88
strangulation, feeling of 26
stress 29, 31–2, 38, 40, 41–2
   cortisol and 119
   school examinations 246–7
sugar 123
sulphur dioxide 213, 215
surgical operations 179
sweat test 65
swimming 205, 239
Symbicort 81, 267
symptoms 16, 24–8
   diary chart 48, *49*
   getting rid of 26
   long-term outlook 219–22
   monitoring 43
   at night 89, 174–5
   remission 16, 163, 244–5
   resembling chest infection 91
   respiratory 44
   returning after long remission
      period 245
   reversibility of 64

symptoms ( *continued*)
system for review of 138
    urgent need for advice 265
    variability 8, 16
    **warning signs of attack**
        251–3
    worse at night 24–5, 47
    worsening 121
    *see also* treatment
syrup 122, 233
tablets *see* steroids, tablets
Tagamet 121
tartrazine (E numbers 102-110
        and 210-219) 215, 293*g*
teachers *see* school
teeth 119, 123
temperature
    air 175, 176
    body 175
terbutaline 83, 112, 141, 145
    in competitive sports 208
    **emergency situations** 255
        away from home 161, 204
    not working 255
    before sexual intercourse 185
    side effects 113
    when to take 82, 91
tests
    for atopy 63–4
    blood tests 64, 73, 121, 238
    blowing tests *see* PEF
    bone densitometry 192
    in diagnosis 50–8
    electrocardiogram (ECG) 221
    exercise testing 59
    heel prick test 65
    reversibility testing 59
    skin prick tests 35, 63–4, 73,
        136, 238, 292*g*

sweat test 65
    therapeutic 233
theophyllines 76, 121, 238, 293*g*
therapeutic test 233
throat 26, 91, 116–17, 119–20
thrush, of mouth or throat 91,
        116–17, 119–20, 293*g*
thunderstorms 211
tickly cough 252
tightness of chest 24, 25, 35, 221,
        226, 255–6
Tilade 80, 83, 166, 237
Timoptol 94
tingling of skin 264
tiredness 28, 38
tobacco *see* smoking
topical steroids 293*g*
    *see also* steroids, inhaled
toys, soft 74–5
trachea (windpipe) *9*, 9, 26, 231,
        293*g*
trade unions 196
travel 198–200, 203–4
treatment
    affecting immune system 120
    altering 162–7
    anti-immunoglobulin E 125–6
    attack when no medication
        available 261–3
    before asthma has developed
        232–3
    combination treatments 81
    cost to NHS 171–2, 218
    of coughs 177–8
    dangers of drug treatments 121
    desensitizing 72
    getting it right first time 128
    holistic approach 77
    how long to continue 163

how to know whether it is
     working 141–2, 168
importance of regularity 82,
     82–3, 85, 89, 91–2
injections 115, 125–6
non-medicine 69–79
not addictive 114
overdosing 237–8
PEF as guide to adjustment
     153
for period pain 187
during pregnancy 188–9
if relievers needed every day
     114
in school hours 240–1
specialization in 139
stopping 163–4, 166–8
when to take 91
see also complementary
     therapies; drugs; inhalers;
     side effects
tree pollen 28, 93–4
trembling or shaking of hands 113
triggers 12, 13, 28–40, 35, 46, 48–9,
     293g
  avoiding 143
  v. causes 29–30
  discovering your triggers 34–5
  reducing exposure to 44
  smoking see smoking
  strenuous exercise 172–3
  variation between individuals
     35, 38, 48
  see also individual triggers
tuberculosis (TB) 66–7
TUC 194, 298
Turbohaler 89, 102, 103, 200
  Braille markings 278
Twisthaler 103, 103, 200

twitchy airways 11, 15–16, 20, 32,
     293g
  inherited element 20–1
  women and 182, 191
types of asthma 59–60

UK Sport 298
uncontrolled asthma 84, 119, 123,
     124, 221, 239, 293g
  complementary therapies and
     75
  recognising 128, 140–5, 250
  seeking medical advice 260,
     266
  signs of 143, 145, 153, 175
  see also control of asthma
Uniphyllin 121
unpredictability of asthma
     attacks 40, 41, 142–3
upper respiratory tract infection
     (URTI) 293g
  see also colds
urbanization 209
urine, difficulty in passing 113
urticaria 42, 62, 214

vacuum cleaners 70–1
ventilation, at work 193
Ventolin 80, 83, 86, 89, 112, 145,
     178
  v. Becotide 84–5
  child's ability to judge dose
     234–6
  in competitive sports 208
  emergency situations 114,
     255, 261–2, 262, 262–4
  away from home 204
  before exercise 206
  increasing need for 141–2

Ventolin (*continued*)
  no effect on osteoporosis 118
  not regularly 115
  not working 255
  side effects 113
  syrup 122
  use only when you have
    symptoms 114
  when breastfeeding 190
  when to take 82, 91, 114, 115
Ventolin Accuhaler 236
Ventolin Evohaler 82, 144, 161
video on asthma 276
viral associated wheeze (VAW) 60
viruses and viral infections 11–12,
    27, 35, 38, 47, 91, 231, 233–4,
    293–4*g*
  as most common cause of
    asthma 28, 92
  *see also* colds
voice problems 116
Voltarol 33
Volumatic 104, *105*, *108*, 116
  for high doses 120, 121, 144
  when breastfeeding 190
vomiting 115, 234, 266–7

walking 192
warning signs of attack 250,
    251–3
  action to take 255–65
wasp sting allergy 72
weather 32, 209–12
websites 295–9
weight loss in children 239
wheezing 11, 24, 25, 31, 35, 47, 211
  in children 31, 60, 226

cold air 32
  in infants 233–4
  not heard 25–6, 254
  as reaction to trigger 175–6
  *see also* silent chest
Windmill trainer for PEF use 155
windpipe (trachea) *9*, 9, 26, 231
wine 213
women
  with asthma 171
  smoking 181–2
wood burning 209
wood dusts 36, 195
work 193–7
  occupations to avoid 194–5
work-aggravated asthma 13, 29,
    44, 193, 196
workplace 29, 171, 183–4
  choosing employment 197
  conditions affecting asthma
    193
  industrial compensation 195
  jobs associated with asthma
    136–7
  smoking in 183–4, 193, 196
  substances causing asthma
    195
World Anti-Doping Agency 208,
    299

Xolair 126

yeast products 215
yoga 77
yoghurt 117
young people *see* adolescents;
    children; puberty

- Asthma UK is the charity dedicated to improving the health and well-being of the 5.2 million people in the UK with asthma.

- Asthma UK works together with people with asthma, healthcare professionals and researchers to develop and share expertise to help people with asthma to increase their understanding of asthma and reduce its effect on their lives.

- Every year we spend around £3 million on research grants and fellowships, each focused on understanding more about asthma, and improving the lives of people with asthma.

- Asthma UK provides support and services for people with asthma including booklets and factfiles with independent, specialist information on every aspect of asthma. The Asthma UK Adviceline provides confidential help and advice from asthma nurse specialists.

If you would like to get the latest information on asthma treatments and care, you can become a member of Asthma UK by simply filling in the form overleaf and returning it to us at the address shown.

### Getting in touch with Asthma UK

**Asthma UK Adviceline: 08457 01 02 03**
*Ask an asthma nurse specialist.*

**Website: asthma.org.uk/adviceline**
*Read the latest advice and news on asthma.*

**Asthma UK publications**
Tel: 020 7786 5000
Email: info@asthma.org.uk
*Request booklets and factfiles on any aspect of asthma.*

**ASTHMA UK, Summit House, 70 Wilson Street, London EC2A 2DB**
REGISTERED CHARITY NUMBER 802364

Yes, I want to get all the latest information on asthma treatments and care by becoming a member of Asthma UK for just £12 a year. As a member of Asthma UK you will receive Asthma Magazine four times a year. Each issue is packed with interviews with people living with asthma, hints on how you can control your symptoms, and features on new research that is helping to improve the lives of people with asthma.

*You can save time and money by calling our Supporter & Information Team on 020 7786 5000 to become a member over the telephone.*

*Alternatively you can set up a standing order by simply completing the form below. Membership costs £12 a year but many people support our work further by paying more.*

## STANDING ORDER FORM

Please pay Asthma UK the sum of £ _____ on the _____ day of _____ and afterwards on the same day. (*Please make this day at least a month from today's date*)

☐ monthly  ☐ quarterly  ☐ annually (until further notice and please debit my account accordingly)

Mr/Mrs/Miss/Ms/Dr/Other _____  First name _____

Surname _____

Address _____

Postcode _____

Telephone _____  Email _____

Account holder's name _____

Bank account number ☐☐☐☐☐☐☐☐

Bank sort code ☐☐☐☐☐☐

Bank name _____

Bank address _____

Postcode _____

Signature _____

### OFFICE USE ONLY

**Instructions to Bank or Building Society:**

Please pay Asthma UK, A/C 36254193, 60-80-07, National Westminster Bank plc, Tavistock Square, London WC1H 9XA -- quoting reference

☐☐☐☐☐☐☐☐☐☐☐☐☐☐☐

*Please return your completed form to*
**FREEPOST RLUR-HJUK-JCEE**
**ASTHMA UK, Summit House, 70 Wilson Street, London EC2A 2DB**

*At Asthma UK we like to keep our members updated about our work and opportunities to support us.*
*If you do not wish us to retain your details, please tick this box* ☐

[AAYF05]

Have you found **Asthma – the 'at your fingertips' guide** useful and practical? If so, you may be interested in other books from Class Publishing.

## COPD
**– the 'at your fingertips' guide**   £14.99
*Dr Jon Miles and June Roberts*
This practical book answers hundreds of real questions asked by people with COPD and their families in plain English, It is easy to understand and tells you what you can do to live your life to the full while living with COPD.

 'The book is excellent and I wish you every success with it.'
 *Dr A C Miller, Consultant Physician, Mayday University Hospital, Croydon*

## Heart Health
**– the 'at your fingertips' guide**   £14.99
*Dr Graham Jackson*
This practical handbook, written by a leading cardiologist, answers all your questions about heart conditions. It tells you all about you and your heart; how to keep your heart healthy, or if it has been affected by heart disease – how to make it as strong as possible.

 'Those readers who want to know more about the various treatments for heart disease will be much enlightened.'
 *Dr James Le Fanu*, Daily Telegraph

## Diabetes
**– the 'at your fingertips' guide**   £14.99
*Professor Peter Sönksen, Dr Charles Fox and Sue Judd*
This is an invaluable reference guide for people with diabetes, which offers practical advice on every aspect of living with the condition, giving you the knowledge and reassurance you need to deal confidently with your diabetes.

 'I have no hesitation in commending this book.'
 *Sir Steve Redgrave CBE, Vice President, Diabetes UK*

## Kidney Dialysis and Transplants
**– the 'at your fingertips' guide**   £14.99
*Dr Andy Stein and Janet Wild with Juliet Auer*
A practical handbook for anyone with long-term kidney failure or their families. The book contains answers to over 450 real questions actually asked by people with end-stage renal failure, and offers positive, clear and medically accurate advice on every aspect of living with the condition.

 'A first class book on kidney dialysis and transplants that is simple and accurate, and can be used to equal advantage by doctors and their patients.'
 *Dr Thomas Stuttaford*, The Times

## High Blood Pressure
**– the 'at your fingertips' guide**   £14.99
*Dr Tom Fahey, Professor Deirdre Murphy with Dr Julian Tudor Hart*
The authors use all their years of experience as blood pressure experts to answer your questions on high blood pressure, in order to give you the information you need to bring your blood pressure down – and keep it down.

 'Readable and comprehensive information.'
 *Dr Sylvia McLaughlan, Director General, The Stroke Association*

## Beating Depression
**– the 'at your fingertips' guide**   £17.99
*Dr Stefan Cembrowicz and Dr Dorcas Kingham*
Depression is one of the most common illnesses in the world – affecting up to one in four people at some time in their lives. *Beating Depression* shows sufferers and their families that they are not alone, and offers tried and tested techniques for overcoming depression.

# PRIORITY ORDER FORM

*Cut out or photocopy this form and send it (post free in the UK) to:*

**Class Publishing**
**FREEPOST 16705**
**Macmillan Distribution**
**Basingstoke**
**RG21 6ZZ**

**Tel: 01256 302 699**
**Fax: 01256 812 558**

**Please send me urgently**
*(tick boxes below)*

*Post included*
*price per copy (UK only)*

☐ **Asthma – the 'at your fingertips' guide**                                     £20.99
(ISBN 10: 1859591116 / ISBN 13: 9781859591116)

☐ **COPD – the 'at your fingertips' guide**                                       £17.99
(ISBN 10: 1859590454 / ISBN 13: 9781859590454)

☐ **Heart Health – the 'at your fingertips' guide**                               £17.99
(ISBN 10: 1859590977 / ISBN 13: 9781859590973)

☐ **Diabetes – the 'at your fingertips' guide**                                   £17.99
(ISBN 10: 185959087X / ISBN 13: 9781859590874)

☐ **Kidney Dialysis and Transplants – the 'at your fingertips' guide**            £17.99
(ISBN 10: 1859590462 / ISBN 13: 9781859590641)

☐ **High Blood Pressure – the 'at your fingertips' guide**                        £17.99
(ISBN 10: 185959090X / ISBN 13: 9781859590904)

☐ **Beating Depression – the 'at your fingertips' guide**                         £20.99
(ISBN 10: 1859591507 / ISBN 13: 9781859591147)

TOTAL _____

## Easy ways to pay

**Cheque:** I enclose a cheque payable to Class Publishing for £ _____

**Credit card:** Please debit my   ☐ Mastercard   ☐ Visa   ☐ Amex

Number _____ Expiry date _____

Name _____

My address for delivery is _____

Town _____ County _____ Postcode _____

Telephone number *(in case of query)* _____

Credit card billing address if different from above _____

Town _____ County _____ Postcode _____

*Class Publishing's guarantee: remember that if, for any reason, you are not satisfied with these books, we will refund all your money, without any questions asked. Prices and VAT rates may be altered for reasons beyond our control.*